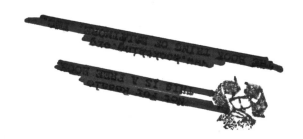

THE COMPLETE GUIDE TO
NATURAL
SLEEP

THE COMPLETE GUIDE TO
NATURAL SLEEP

. . . . .

Dian Dincin Buchman, Ph.D.

GRAMERCY BOOKS
NEW YORK

This 2003 edition is published by Gramercy Books, an imprint of Random House Value Publishing, a division of Random House, Inc., New York, by arrangement with Keats Publishing, a division of NTC/Contemporary Publishing Group, Inc., Lincolnwood, Illinois.

Gramercy is a registered trademark and the colophon is a trademark of Random House, Inc.

Random House
New York • Toronto • London • Sydney • Auckland
www.randomhouse.com

Printed in the United States of America

Library of Congress Cataloging-in-Publication Data

Buchman, Dian Dincin.
    The complete guide to natural sleep / Dian Dincin Buchman.
        p. cm.
    Previously published: New Canaan, Conn. : Keats Pub., 1997.
    Includes bibliographical references and index.
    ISBN 0-517-22238-8
    1. Sleep—Popular works. 2. Sleep disorders—Popular works. I. Title.

RA786 .B83 2003
616.8'498—dc21

                                                    2002037947

9 8 7 6 5 4 3 2 1

*To my favorite person in all the world,
my daughter Caitlin,
one of the world's great sleepers.*

Acknowledgments

I am indebted to many people for their support, ideas, information and encouragement, especially Caitlin Kraft Buchman and Tanya Adler.

My thanks to the following people for providing specialized sleep information: Gregory Mader of the American Sleep Disorders Association; Morgan Hughes, staff coordinator, Emory Sleep Disorders Center; Phyllis Herman, Keats Publishing; Karen Di Bernardo; Jeffery B. Blumberg, Ph.D.

Sleep is a profound, complex specialty, and I am greatly indebted to the research, comments and views of the following sleep experts: Donald Bliwise, M.D., Richard Ferber, M.D., Peter J. Hauri, Ph.D., Professor Peretz Lavie, Ph.D., Ronald E. Dahl, M.D., Virgil Wooten, M.D., Sonia Ancoli-Israel, Ph.D., Mark Rosekind, Ph.D., Wallace Mendelson, M.D., Mary Carskadon, Ph.D., Amy R. Wolfson, Ph.D., Jerry Rosen, M.D., Richard Wurtman, M.D., William Dement, M.D., Ph.D., Timothy Monk, Ph.D., Deepak Chopra, M.D.

I thank the following people for sharing interesting sleep stories and/or sleep experiences: Betty Sue Eaton, Caitlin Kraft Buchman, Ann Reit, Jerry Dincin, Barbara Rubin, Ph.D., Elyse Sommer, Judge Jarred Siegal, Barbara Seaman, Jane Wilson, Arnold Nash, Nena O'Neil, Zola Dincin Schneider, Michael Richards, Rose Robbins, Thomas Culhane, Judy Feiffer, Cynthia Medalie, Doe Lang, Ph.D., Jonathan Thorpe, Janice LaRouche, Daniel Hales, Barbara Gordon, Alan Pomerantz, Ph.D., Sandra Weiner, Fran Klein, Michael Locke, Ph.D., Costanza Biocco, Catlin Adams, Scott Crawford, Maryann Clarke, Linda Geiser, Helga Shepard, James Griffith, Claire Gerus, Harley Warner, Anne Sellaro, Wallace Cornell, Pierre Van Meenen, Lynn Bien.

I want to thank my many friends for their support despite the demands put upon me by multiple projects and Carol Williams of the legal department of the Authors Guild, Robin Rue of the Anita Diamant Agency and my canny Scotsman, Don McKay, Esq.

I thank Norman Goldfind, president of Keats, for arranging for me to attend the Nashville sleep conference; Donald Bensen, editor-in-chief of Keats, for his easy attitude; and my editor, Susan E. Davis, for understanding the significance and thrust of this book.

Contents

THE COMPLETE GUIDE TO
NATURAL SLEEP

Introduction

Sleep is a complex, somewhat mysterious daily activity. It takes about a third of our life and is vital to our mental, physical and emotional health. Everyone has some sleepless intervals. Usually they pass. However, millions of us, in fact, about a third of the world's population, develop long-standing periods of desperate sleeplessness. Whether it is of short duration or a long-standing pattern, insomnia can be caused by life stresses which provoke anxiety, excess caffeine, the inability to relax, poor sleeping habits, side effects of medication or a physical illness that causes distracting pain.

Although sleep and dreams have been observed for thousands of years, we still don't have an absolute answer about why we sleep. However, we know a lot more about sleep since a breakthrough laboratory observation in the 1950s when it was noted that a baby's eyes *moved* during sleep. That simple revelation became the cornerstone of all subsequent investigations into the nature of sleep. Eventually it led to the knowledge that sleep is divided into different cycles of dreaming and nondreaming. No one can survive without dreamtime; nor can we live or be healthy without nondreaming time. Both are essential for our well-being and restoration. The different stages and the meaning of each stage of sleep are explained for both adults and children in this book.

Expanding numbers of people are uneasy about taking synthetic drugs for illness and insomnia because they are concerned about the many deleterious side effects. That accounts for a yearning for and growing awareness of preventive answers and natural solutions to all health questions. To answer this thirst for knowledge, I have sought out sleep research from around the globe to discover the many common-sense and natural remedy answers presented here. While this book leans strongly on the official self-help procedures offered by careful sleep scientists, it also presents a wide range of other safe natural remedies and sleep strategies culled from cutting-edge nutritional information and the best of ancient and modern plant-based medicine and water therapies that all promote good sleep.

This book includes a thorough-going discussion of sleep needs and natural solutions for all ages and is divided into three parts. The first part is devoted to adults, ranging from the young adult through advanced older age. Four chapters cover how we sleep; typical causes of insomnia, such as aging, certain foods, jet lag and conditions like pregnancy and meno-pause; positive sleep strategies, such as helpful sleep habits, foods and supplements; and natural sleep remedies organized into an at-a-glance problem and solution chart.

Special attention is devoted in Part I to such topics as:

- Food and nutrition: Substances that cause sleeplessness are identified, as are foods that affect moods and promote sleep.
- Melatonin: This natural substance can be taken in very low dosages to combat jet lag, promote alertness during shift work and just get a good night's sleep.
- Light: Sleep scientists have developed light therapies to overcome inappropriate sleep patterns, help shift workers adjust to their hours and prevent winter depression.

The second part of the book is devoted to children. Three chapters cover infants, toddlers and school children, and teens special sleep prob-lems. Each includes recent laboratory research, a unique section of scenar-ios (scripts) which parents can use to cure common sleep difficulties, a broad variety of step-by-step natural remedies and at-a-glance problem and solution charts. All chapters contain simple, practical strategies and behav-ior modification recommendations to overcome the most common types of children's sleep problems.

The third part of the book includes the following safe, nondrug, natural therapies to achieve sleep:

- Plants: Soothing and relaxing herbs can be used in three ways: inter-nally as teas or pills and externally either in foot or full baths or as poultices or compresses.
- Homeopathy: Homeopathic remedies, tissue salts and Bach flower remedies promote sleep and end sleep disturbances.
- Water: Direct and indirect water modalities can effortlessly ease you off to sleep.
- Stretching exercises: Simple physical exercises relax the body, making it easier to sleep.
- Finger pressure or acupressure: Using ancient Asian wisdom, you can press specific points on the body to help promote sleep.

- Mental imagery and meditation: Visualization techniques help circumvent insomnia and even allow you to use your brain to solve problems while you sleep.

As the great German philosopher Friedrich Nietzsche said, "No small art is it to sleep: it is necessary for that purpose to keep awake all day." May this book help you awake each morning refreshed and ready to live life to the fullest.

PART

I

Adult Sleep Problems and Solutions

Sleep disorders and insomnia are problems among young and old throughout the world. But some conditions can have more serious consequences than others. For instance, Dr. J.V., a Denver anesthesiologist was tried for falling asleep during minor surgery in which an 8-year-old boy died. John Rogers in California is an example of what the American Medical Association calls "America's hidden nightmare." He is one of 1,500 people a year who end up in fatal driving accidents due to sleep deprivation.

A scientific approach to sleep only started in the 1950s and is considered a truly new science. One of the world's pioneer sleep researchers, William C. Dement, M.D., Ph.D., Director of the Sleep Disorders Clinic and Laboratory at Stanford University School of Medicine, stresses the importance of a decent night's sleep when he says, "Lack of sleep can lead to a poor performance at work. Sleep-deprived individuals have more difficulty remembering things, thinking logically, understanding spoken instructions and making decisions—all of which are essential contributors to job performance." While researchers know a lot about how we sleep, they still can't agree on why we sleep. Some claim it is mainly to achieve energy, others to restore the body, while some insist on a combination of rejuvenation as well as energy. More research is needed before we know conclusively why human beings need to spend about a third of their lifetime asleep.

Since sleep is absolutely necessary to survival and good health, many researchers are alarmed because throughout the world, from adolescence to older adulthood, people are getting less sleep than they did in past decades. This was confirmed in an article in the journal *Sleep* [19(6):462–464(1996)], in which Donald Bliwise, Ph.D., the director of the Sleep Disorders Center at Emory University Medical School in Atlanta, found that today's adults usually don't get enough sleep to feel good and function well the next day. Bliwise evaluated past and present sleep habits by questioning 1,200 healthy adults ranging from 18 to past 70 and comparing his questionnaires with data published from the 1930s onward.

Bliwise learned that every decade since the 1930s has shown a decrease in sleeptime. Healthy working adults in a 1959 study said they slept 6 to 7 hours a night; similar adults polled in the mid-1980s slept about one hour less. College students in a 1988 study reported sleeping about 30 minutes less than college students did in 1978. Bliwise points out today's Americans are also spending more time at work. In the twenty years from 1969 to 1989 they increased the time spent at work by 153 hours a year. This "volunteer" work ethic shows a sharp increase during the nineties.

The World Health Organization (WHO) called a worldwide sleep conference in September 1995. Among the participants were 15 countries, including the American Sleep Disorders Association and the Sleep Research Society. The WHO group report noted that one in four adults around the world is so sleep-deprived that they have trouble falling asleep or staying asleep, and they do not perceive sleep to be refreshing or restorative. America ranks high in insomnia, with one-third of adults claiming some nightly disturbance and one in ten adults describing serious and persistent sleep difficulties. The National Commission on Sleep Disorders Research tallied the direct costs of insomnia in the United States as exceeding $15 billion annually. However, according to Thomas Roth, Ph.D, Division Head of the Henry Ford Health System Sleep Disorders and Research Center in Detroit and one of the authors of the WHO report, this vast sum does not cover lost workdays, pain, suffering, accidents or loss of life. "These indirect costs may be greater than the direct costs," says Dr. Roth.

Insomniacs spend hours every night in worried anticipation that they will not fall asleep or get back to sleep if awakened. They report feeling less well physically and less able to enjoy contact with family and friends. They also complain about memory lapses and difficulties in concentrating during daytime sleepiness. The National Institute of Mental Health found people who said they had insomnia had a higher risk of later developing a major depressive disorder than those who slept adequately. More than half the insomniacs studied worldwide by WHO had problems with anxiety, depression or alcohol. (Four in ten insomniacs have tried alcohol or over-the-counter medi-

Causes of Adult Insomnia

One in every two adults reports having some trouble sleeping. The most common causes include:

- Job-related stress.
- Financial worries.
- Family crises.
- Unsettling interruptions from babies, toddlers and school-age children.
- Inability to sleep because nighttime jobs make it hard to sleep during the daytime.
- Medical problems: pain, arthritis and asthma attacks are among the reasons cited by people over 55 years of age.

---

cations to help them sleep better.) Auto accidents are twice as widespread in people who claim insomnia than those who feel they sleep well.

However, the sense of not getting enough sleep is sometimes a matter of personal perception. Some people who considered themselves poor sleepers, when tested throughout the night in a sleep laboratory, turned out to have average sleep habits. Canadian Stephen Leacock tells how when he was young, he and his brother complained to each other about not sleeping: "When I was a young man living in a boarding house in Toronto, my brother George came to visit me, and since there was no spare room, we had to share my bed. In the morning, after daylight, I said to George, 'Did you get much sleep?' 'Not a damn minute,' said he. 'Neither did I,' I rejoined. 'I could hear every sound all night.' Then we put our heads up from the bedclothes and saw that the bed was covered with plaster. The ceiling had fallen down on us in the night, but we hadn't noticed it. We had 'insomnia.' "

Research indicates some people sleep fairly well until they reach their 40s, 50s or 60s, and then, seemingly for no apparent reason, patterns change and sleep becomes more elusive. That leads many people to believe the need for sleep evaporates as one gets older, but research shows if you needed 6 hours at 40, you'll still need 6 hours at 77. If you craved a full 8 hours of sleep when you were younger, you'll need the same amount at 55 and at 80. It doesn't mean you'll get the amount you need, but your body will require it.

Laboratory studies of sleep habits indicate that changes in sleep occur as people age. The lighter, more easily arousable stages of sleep increase, while the restorative and deeper stages of sleep decrease. To avoid this downward spiral, researchers urge patients to exercise several times a week and to find mentally challenging interests. They point out that except for medically caused insomnia (such as narcolepsy and sleep apnea), the sleeplessness we call insomnia is quite responsive to a wide variety of drug-free, self-help methods such as behavior modification and routines that are generally called "sleep hygiene."

How We Sleep

Sleep is not one continuous, seamless accomplishment, nor is it a closing down of body functions. Though you are not aware of it while you sleep, there are two types of sleep: REM and nonREM (NREM). REM refers to rapid-eye-movement sleep in which the eyes actually dart about under closed eyelids. REM is dreaming sleep, which in adults occurs about every ninety minutes during the night. NREM is conventional, nondreaming sleeptime, when the eyes do not dart around.

Dreaming during REM sleep takes place intermittently during the night. This sleep has some qualities of a wakeful state: not only do the eyes move about, but the heartbeat accelerates, then decelerates, blood pressure rises and falls and muscles quiver and twitch. REM sleep lasts between five to fifteen minutes. Usually, the first REM period lasts for a few minutes, and then they gradually lengthen during the night, for a total of about one and a half hours. The longest dream period occurs just before waking up. This dreamtime averages between 20 and 25 percent of our sleeptime.

NREM sleep accounts for about three quarters of the time we sleep. It has four separate transitional stages, each one a little deeper. Stage 1 is the gradual drifting from an awake state to a light sleeping state, a twilight zone between awareness and sleep, from which one is easily awakened. Breathing and pulse become more level and the muscles relax. Stages 2 and 3 are transitional stages which lead into the fourth stage of very deep sleep (called "delta sleep"). In stage 2, breathing and heart rate slow down. During stage 3 the body temperature falls, blood pressure is lowered and breathing and heart rate continue to slow down.

Stage 4 is the deepest and the most restorative sleep phase. The very first plummet into deep sleep lasts about an hour for a young healthy adult. In stage 4 nature has seen to it that the body is almost paralyzed and that we are not responsive to outside stimuli, with the exception of such crisis sounds as emergency calls of distress, fire or the sound of one's child crying. In this deep fourth stage, which is the most restorative, it is almost as if the mind and body are drifting in a huge enveloping cloud, but the cloud has one gap of light through which the conscious mind stays on the alert. The body restores itself, repairs bone, muscle and skin tissues and acts like a "fountain of youth" during deep, nondreaming sleeptime.

These four stages of NREM sleep constantly repeat themselves after REM episodes. Actually, patterns of long NREM/REM sleep cycles recur continually throughout the night. When stage 4 ends, we move automatically into REM time, when the closed eyes dart about as if watching a motion picture, but what we are watching is really our dreams.

Many key sleep researchers believe people need the dream period to sort out the events of the day and to place information into the brain's memory bank. "Dreaming permits each and every one of us to be quietly and safely insane every night of our lives," says Dr. William Dement, M.D., Ph.D., director of the Sleep Disorders Clinic and Laboratory at Stanford University School of Medicine. Most people "catch" the dream details about once a week, although women routinely recall more dreams than men. However, that also depends on whether or not you tend to wake up during a dream cycle. Nightmares that wake you with a small "jump" or start tend to be remembered.

From times immemorial there have been communities and civilizations that conjured up different uses and interpretations of the dream state. The early Greeks used dream analysis to heal mental and physical states. A more primitive society, the Senoi, used reconstruction of dreams and dream discussions to redraw bad dreams into positive ones. These days, many people successfully practice modern versions of Senoi constructive

Sleep and Memory

Even after one has spent a lot of time memorizing a list or certain physical actions or solved a specific mathematical problem, one needs a complete night of sleep to consolidate and fix the material in the memory. For instance, according to a report in the April 1996 *Canadian Medical Association Journal*, any loss of REM dream sleep affects thinking and memory tasks ("cognitive procedural tasks"). Physical (motor) tasks such as a gym routine, remembering Tai Chi or yoga movements or what to do on the football field are affected by loss of light sleep that occurs early in the morning.

dreaming, and constructive dream experts show us how the sleeping brain can be used during the night to analyze and solve problems as if it were a huge mainline computer (see Chapter 10).

A Hidden Clock Determines Our Sleep Patterns

Deep in the recesses of the brain is a tiny regulator, an internal clock, known as the "circadian rhythm," which tells you when you are sleepy and when you should get up. This internal biological clock can change the body's rhythm and advance or delay the sleep-wake cycle. Like an unruly pendulum on a grandfather clock, most hard-to-manage sleep problems are actually the result of an out-of-sync internal clock. A character in Evelyn Waugh's *Decline and Fall* complains, "I haven't been to sleep for over a year. That's why I go to bed early. One needs more rest if one doesn't sleep."

All living things—even one-celled plants and animals (the two possible exceptions may be viruses and bacteria)—have an internal means of measuring time. These innate clocks regulate the living thing's natural rhythms—times of activity and rest—that allow a plant to open to the sun and an animal to be alert during the time when its prey is available. These clocks also regulate the sequence in the being's development. For example, the mechanism ensures that a plant will grow roots before flowers and a newborn baby won't grow teeth before it has a fully matured stomach. Biological clocks are linked to the seasons. Deciduous trees, for example, grow leaves during the lengthening days of spring and drop them when daylight shortens in autumn. Migrating birds depend on their biological clocks, in addition to navigational references to the sun and stars, to guide them across huge distances. These rhythms have been known to naturalists for centuries. The great 18th-century Swedish botanist Carolus Linnaeus even grew a garden that told time—he planted flowers so that they opened and closed their blossoms an hour apart around the clock! However, scientists still don't know whether the biological clock is a single master mechanism or a number of interrelated rhythms. Because these rhythms have a frequency that's about, but not exactly, twenty-four hours, they have been called "circadian" rhythms from the Latin for "about" (*circa*) and "daily" (*dies*).

Each person is born with his own innate rhythm. In some people a pattern of being owls or larks emerges in childhood and persists throughout our lives. Larks and owls live and sleep at opposite parts of the day and night. Many

Five Stages of Sleep

Each sleep cycle lasts about ninety minutes each night. People have four to six such cycles depending on how long they sleep. However, the important consideration is not the number of cycles but how much continuous comfortable sleep one gets.

Stage	What's Happening	Time Element	Special/Dream Facts	Eyes	Brain Cells	Muscles	Heart	Temperature	Misc.
STAGE ONE: Transition sleep (drowsiness)	In bed, muscles relax, mind drifts like going down a staircase; drift into stage 2.	1/2 min. to several minutes.	Gliding, floating feeling, dreams and thoughts drift as on clouds; easily roused.	Move about under closed eyelids.	Go on standby, some parts asleep, others not; awareness of external world lessens.	Relaxed.	Slows down.	Falls.	Sugar increases in bloodstream.
STAGE TWO: Light Sleep	Drift into stage 3.	Varies.	Drowsy state like day dreaming; imagery similar to later dream state.	Not seeing; if eyes open, may roll from side to side.	Short bursts of rapid activity and slow waves.	Sometimes a fleeting quiver of the body wakes you briefly.	Decrease in blood pressure.	Falls.	Can be awakened easily.

STAGE THREE	Fall more deeply asleep; transition into stage 4.	Deep sleep; not aware of outside world.	Brain waves get slower.		Rate gets more stable.	Slightly harder to awaken.
STAGE FOUR: Deep (delta) sleep	Delta sleep (deep physical repose): recovery, recuperation.	If delta sleep is missed, you wake up feeling weary.	Brain can think, but thinking is splintered; brain waves slow.	Body lies very still because brain is not sending messages to muscles to move; muscles even more relaxed than when awake.	Regulation impaired; do not sweat or shiver.	Breathing stable; hard to arouse, but if stimulus is dire, can process some information.

Five Stages of Sleep (continued)

Stage	What's Happening	Time Element	Special/ Dream Facts	Eyes	Brain Cells	Muscles	Heart	Temperature	Misc.
REM/ DREAM SLEEP	Body uses more oxygen.		Respond to signals from within your own body instead of outside world; can accept outlandish nature of dreams. If awakened after REM, will always report a dream.	Bursts of rapid eye movements.	Elevated blood pressure & heavier flow to brain; brain waves look like combination of drowsiness & waking.	Tone greatly depleted; significant relaxation of head & neck; body seems to be paralyzed except for eyes, breathing, hearing & penile erections.	Rate elevated and irregular.		Elevated rate of breathing; possible psychological function: to process emotional experiences & transfer recent memories into long-term storage.

a marriage has suffered because of conflicting inner schedules, and it takes great gifts of accommodation and independence for larks and owls to coexist. Strangely, even lark adolescents can become owls temporarily during their teen years. Many mature adults become larks as they grow older. They go to bed at an unseemly early hour and get up in the middle of the night. The chances are strong that their internal clocks need to be "reset."

Basic reconditioning techniques work well in the case of a "disordered" internal clock, and troubled sleepers do well when supervised by knowledgeable sleep experts. Often making some simple lifestyle changes helps, such as creating a regular nightly sleep ritual or routine, eliminating caffeine-based foods, drinks and prescriptions from the diet after noon or avoiding an alcohol nightcap, which may lead to fragmented sleep and groggy awakenings.

A Lark Outsmarts an Owl

Making sure, by all means, that you get the sleep you need is the moral of the famous story of the 13th-century painter Buffamacco, a lark, and his year of nighttime hell. Buffamacco moved next door to a successful woolworker without realizing he would never get a wink of sleep because the woolworker's wife, an owl, worked all night at her spinning wheel. The wheel made a terrible racket and kept the painter up when he wanted to sleep. After about a year of not sleeping, the painter became desperate.

When he noticed that there was a small hole between their adjoining buildings and that the hole opened over his neighbor's cooking pot, he hollowed out his cane, and each evening shoved it through the wall, dropping a quarter of a cup of salt in the woolworker's evening meal. After a series of inedible meals the rich woolworker began to loudly berate his wife for her terrible cooking. Her irate screams brought a number of alarmed neighbors, including the unsurprised Buffamacco to their door. The woolworker desperately explained the cause of his distress.

Buffamacco offered a new approach, "You complain that the pot is too much salted, but I marvel that this good woman can do anything well, considering that the whole night she sits up over that wheel of hers and has not an hour's sleep. Let her give up this all-night work and sleep, so she will have her wits about her by day and will not fall into such blunders."

The woolworker accepted Buffamacco's advice, and from that time onward the painter enjoyed undisturbed sleep.

How the Hormone Melatonin Influences Sleep

Typically, hormone production, body temperature and other biological activities come and go on a regular twenty-four hour schedule regulated by the circadian rhythm. Fluctuations of these substances are actually governed by the pea-sized pineal gland deep within the brain, following the orders of the internal clock. One of this gland's several functions is to gently secrete melatonin, a hormone which serves as nature's timekeeper. This delivery of melatonin has its own normal rhythm, which is dependent on various light and darkness cues keyed to the rotation of the earth. Melatonin is manufactured in darkness, but starts an infinitesimal secretion about dusk and sometime in the early night signals us when to be sleepy and, as it ebbs, when to feel awake. A pioneer melatonin researcher, Dr. Alfred Lewy of the Sleep Disorders Research Section at Oregon Health Sciences University in Portland, helped discover after years of painstaking study how darkness encourages and light inhibits the manufacture of this time-cueing substance.

What is known is that infants and older children sleep so much because they produce high amounts of melatonin. Such secretion lessens as we age, and this fact has caused a variety of sleep researchers to automatically assume the lack of melatonin is a prime cause of sleep irregularities among mature adults. However, Dr. Lewy strongly disagrees with this premise. Not only does the amount and timing of melatonin production vary from person to person, Lewy believes the primary function of melatonin is to readjust errant internal clocks.

After long years of investigation by sleep researchers, pharmaceutical houses started manufacturing animal and synthetic duplicates of melatonin. Some produce it from the pineal glands of cows, others by chemical replication. As I write, there is a virtual stampede of consumers using melatonin for the management of sleep and jet lag; others are using it because of all the hype that melatonin is a youth pill. I've done my own polling on the use of this hormone while talking with a wide variety of people in various Internet chat rooms. This informal poll corroborates the formal research papers in the field. A substantial group of insomniacs report success with the use of varying amounts for regulation of sleep problems. Melatonin is great for jet lag. Melatonin can be used under supervision by a sleep physician for control of shift work. On the other hand, dozens of others told me either they hadn't the slightest positive reaction to taking melatonin or they had both minor or significant side effects.

Administration of melatonin pills, says Dr. Lewy, can fool the internal body clock into thinking dusk is arriving earlier (or later) or daylight is arriving earlier (or later). In either case, after days, perhaps weeks, or sometimes months of precisely timed and quite low doses, one's body clock eventually comes back to its normal circadian level. Like a grandfather clock pendulum, an adjusted internal body clock gives accurate, normal time and no longer advances or delays itself. Dr. Lewy is quite persuasive in his arguments for the precise timing of melatonin doses since careless application can create a totally opposite effect than that intended. Badly self-dosed insomniacs have been documented at various sleep disorder centers with their internal clocks moved in the wrong direction. For example, the patient might be living in Pittsburgh, but her internal body clock is geared to London. Accurate dosing and spacing of the hormone can avoid this problem.

University researchers who have seen all the positive as well as the negative results of melatonin use urge caution in taking this substance on a daily basis for long periods of time. The general consensus is summed up by Dr. Clifford Singer of the Department of Geriatric Psychiatry in Oregon Health Science University who advises prudence in melatonin use. "It is safe in the short term," he says, "but its long range consequences are not known." (Do not take melatonin supplements without first reading more about the hormone—especially warnings about its use and possible side effects—at the end of Chapter 4.)

Sleep Efficiency Ebbs with Aging

A slow change in sleep patterns occurs between the ages of 20 and 50, with sleep efficiency decreasing in both men and women after 50. As we age, the restorative fourth deep sleep stage is reduced by 50 and 60 percent, and awakenings during the night double and later double once again. Young adults generally awaken between three to five times during a normal night's sleep, but some elderly adults can be aroused as many as 100 times (some say as many as 150 times). Most healthy sleepers forget the awakenings and are immediately able to return to sleep.

Researchers say that sleep efficiency starts to lessen as early as the age of 30 in men. Men's arousal from sleep increases gradually after the age of 40. Women's sleep starts to be seriously challenged by age 50. Both men and women over 70 spend more time in bed, but actually get less sleeptime, because the increase in arousals tends to fragment one's sleep. Sleep investigators agree that most sleep problems can be offset with strong nighttime sleep rituals, consistent exercise and stimulating things to do in the daytime. Preventive disease practitioners also advise a whole series of natural, nondrug remedies that can help most people overcome sleep irregularities (see Part III).

Conditions That Interfere with Sleep

Unfortunately, many things can disrupt a good night's sleep. Some things, such as the foods we eat, are relatively easy to control. Other things like chronic medical conditions or circadian rhythm disturbances can cause considerable havoc before we're able to bring them under control.

Medical Conditions That Aggravate Sleep

Have you ever been awakened by heartburn after eating a heavy meal late at night? Or maybe you've had arthritis pains awaken you from a sound sleep? Unfortunately, a number of medical conditions can keep you awake or even wake you up in the middle of the night. On the other hand, what's keeping you awake might be the medicine you're taking for a medical condition. A variety of coping strategies—all involving natural healing methods (see Chapter 8 for a thorough discussion of herbal remedies, homeopathy and tissue salts)—are provided for the illnesses discussed below.

ALLERGIES

The antihistamines you're taking for allergies may cause drowsiness during the day and insomnia at night.

COPING STRATEGIES: There are many natural herbal, homeopathic and tissue salt remedies for allergy problems. For instance, that ancient Greek concoction oxymel made with apple cider vinegar and honey is often effective. Add either one tablespoon or one teaspoon each of honey and apple cider vinegar to a glass of water. It will taste like tart apple juice. Start drinking this preparation freely two months prior to and all through the allergy season. You can make up large batches and store them in the refrigerator. For best results, make sure the honey and vinegar are organic. This drink also has a calming effect on children over one year of age. (Note: Do not give honey to children under one year of age.)

ANGINA PECTORIS

Angina causes chest pain during the night, which clearly interferes with quality sleep. These pains may lead to additional anxiety and chronic insomnia, which often force a sufferer into dependency on prescription sleeping drugs. Angina also affects sleep by delaying the time it takes to fall asleep. The medicines used for this condition usually also reduce the restorative sleep of stages 3 and 4.

ARTHRITIS

Patients with osteoarthritis that causes inflammation or pain in one or more joints find their pain is usually worse in the late afternoon or evening. If they are awakened by pain, it is usually in the key restorative sleep stages of 2, 3 and 4, and they cannot fall asleep easily again. Rheumatoid arthritis pain is usually worse in the morning.

Coping Strategies: Keeping supple is very important for arthritis patients. Do mild exercise, yoga-type stretching, Tai Chi (a slow Chinese martial art exercise) or Qigung (slow Chinese exercises that also activate and energize the body).
The following are known aids to offset arthritis-based sleep problems:

- Daily intake of oxymel: equal amounts (a teaspoon or tablespoon) of apple cider vinegar and honey in a glass of pure water.
- Hot tubs and hot baths in Epsom salts give comfort.
- Castor oil packs during the day or through the night help alleviate pain.
- Lemon rubs are useful and soothing.
- Homeopathic Arnica ointment can be applied topically to painful joints or take one tablet of 30c/x Arnica for an acute attack during the night. (For a thorough discussion of tissue salts see Chapter 8.

Note that you can buy them in *either* 30c or 30x, which is abbreviated here as 30c/x.) For longer-range therapy, take 6x Arnica under the tongue three times a day for about two weeks at a time.
- In the last few years several companies have put out excellent red pepper-based topical ointments which can greatly relieve pain. The ointment takes about two weeks before it starts to work, but it can be used thereafter on a consistent basis. These are available over-the-counter in pharmacies or health food stores.
- Valerian root in the form of a pill or an extract will quiet the nerves and modify the pain.
- Pineapple or bromelin enzymes protect the body from further free radical damage and also stimulate digestion of protein.

AVOID: Iron pills.

TEST OUT AND POSSIBLY AVOID: Although this varies from one arthritis sufferer to another, a certain percentage of patients are sensitive to foods in the nightshade family. When they eliminate tomatoes, white potatoes, eggplant and green peppers, they often feel a lot better.

ASTHMA AND OTHER CHRONIC BREATHING PROBLEMS

Asthma attacks and other chronic breathing problems occur 100 times more often during the usual hours of sleep than at other times of the day. In *The Principles and Practice of Sleep Medicine*, Dr. Donald Bliwise comments that vast numbers of the elderly (clearly in the millions) show some disturbed breathing problems during sleep. Pulmonary disease causes nighttime spasms which decrease the total time spent in sleep and cause numerous arousals. The usually prescribed nasal sprays, which are central nervous system stimulants, actually worsen insomnia.

COPING STRATEGIES: Dr. Bliwise suggests nonsurgical solutions, including monitoring weight, curbing liquor intake and taking naps. He also recommends investigating the use of continuous positive airway pressure (CPAP) devices obtainable through sleep clinics.

WAYS TO REDUCE NIGHTTIME ASTHMA SYMPTOMS THROUGH INDOOR ALLERGEN CONTROL:
- Use an air conditioner, especially during pollen seasons.
- Keep all the bedding encased in double cotton covers (duvets) to decrease exposure to dust mite allergens.
- Select allergy-free pillows which inhibit mold and mildew growth.

- Do a dust check of the bedroom. What collects dust? Throw away all dust-collecting curtains, books, magazines, carpets, toys and so on.
- Each week kill dust mites by washing all bedding in hot water.
- Frequently vacuum the bedroom. Dust with a damp rag.
- Wash pets frequently. Keep pets out of the bedroom.

HEARTBURN

Heartburn creates a strong acid taste in the mouth and a burning feeling in the chest. These symptoms result from an excess of acid regurgitated from the stomach into the throat. This reflux of acid and pain frequently awakens people from sleep. Many patients reach for a sleeping pill at this point, wanting not to be awakened by the problem. However, the journal *Geriatrics* (no. 41, 1/31/86) describes how unsafe sleeping pills can be for patients with heartburn. If you cannot wake up when a reflux occurs, eventually the acid erodes and inflames the area, causing a painful condition called "reflux esophagitis."

SIDE EFFECTS OF TAKING ANTACIDS: Some people take antacids to stop heartburn. However, specific products have the following side effects:

- Antacids with high doses of hidden aluminum, such as Amphogel and Rolaids, can affect the quality of your sleep. Consistent use of antacids may pile up as many as 1000 mg a day of aluminum so watch those labels. In fact, menopausal women should avoid all products with aluminum.
- Antacids with magnesium, such as Camalox, Gelucil, Maalox, Mylanta and Riopan, may cause diarrhea and, if used frequently, may lower blood pressure, which can cause fainting and/or heartbeat irregularities.
- Antacids with sodium, such as Alka Seltzer and Bromo-Seltzer, are to be avoided if one is on a salt-restricted diet.
- Antacids with calcium, such as Alka-2 and Tums, if taken too frequently, may cause bloating, cramps and constipation.
- Antacids with aspirin side effects may interfere with blood clotting and cause possible ringing in the ears or Reye's syndrome. Pepto-Bismol (bismuth-salicylate) has known aspirin side effects.
- Drugs that change gastric secretions, such as Tagamet, Zantac and others, affect the stomach's ability to overcome alcohol, making the alcohol more potent. Don't take a nightcap if taking these drugs.

COPING STRATEGIES: When heartburn occurs, immediately drink one or more large glasses of water. This cuts the acid and usually works. Many people also respond to an increased intake of pure water and hydrochloric and betaine supplements to replace depleted HCL acid in the stomach which occurs after age 40. It is also possible to restructure your need for antacids by consulting a nutritional counselor.

OTHER HELPFUL TACTICS INCLUDE: Eat small, frequent meals. Do not lie down after eating. When you do lie down, prop pillows around you to make sure you are lying on your left side. The stomach lies lower in your body when you are on your left side and keeps the stomach acid still, which prevents it from migrating to the esophagus. Another age-old solution is to permanently lift the head of your bed with balanced, stable wooden blocks.

HERBAL REMEDIES: To counter the pain of heartburn, slowly sip a teaspoon of apple cider vinegar in a half glass of water. Ginger in cooked food and powdered ginger capsules help sponge up excess stomach acid. Use papaya or bromelain tablets as aids to digestion. Three herbal teas that aid digestion are bruised fennel seed (an anti-inflammatory), peppermint (a calming sedative) and lemon balm (another herbal relaxer).

TISSUE SALTS: The following help with both heartburn and sleeplessness due to digestive problems: The main digestive cell salt aid is Nat. Phos., which acts as an acid neutralizer and against acid dyspepsia; take five 6c/x tablets. To help restore sluggish organs and tissues, take a dose of Calcarea Phos., as it speeds recovery from any acute problem.

AVOID: Using aspirin or caffeine products; being constipated, as straining places undue pressure on the abdomen; smoking, as nicotine contributes to heartburn.

HYPERTENSION

There are two connections between hypertension and sleep. The first, mentioned in the June 1996 issue of *Hypertension*, was that researchers in Japan found that blood pressure rose after a night of insufficient sleep. The second is that many drugs used for hypertension can have an adverse effect on sleep. Beta-blockers, clonidine, reserpine and methyldopa all produce central nervous system activity which can change sleep rhythm and physiology. Diuretics produce unwanted urges to urinate during the night and delays in falling back to sleep.

It's interesting to note that if you're taking drugs for high blood pressure, it's best not to drink grapefruit juice, says Dr. Frederic J. Vagnini in *Cardio-*

vascular Wellness Newsletter. Tests have shown that grapefruit juice may increase or decrease the amount of medication that enters the bloodstream and "may interfere with certain calcium channel blockers that are used to control blood pressure and chest pain—it has been shown to triple the level of this drug in a person's bloodstream. Orange juice appears to have no such effect."

INCONTINENCE

Incontinence, or lack of bladder control, produces a sensation of the need to urinate. Men with prostate problems often experience the same sensation. This results in frequent arousals from sleep.

COPING STRATEGIES: Do not drink any liquids at least one hour before bedtime. Void just before getting into bed.

You can regain bladder control and counteract stress incontinence with biofeedback training and by practicing Kegel exercises: Three times a day practice contraction of the lower part of the body as if holding back urination or stool for at least 10 counts.

TISSUE SALTS (for a thorough discussion of tissue salts see Chapter 8; note that you can buy them in *either* 6c or 6x sizes, which has been abbreviated here as 6c/x):

- Take 6c/x Ferrum Phos. if you have a sudden or frequent urge to urinate; if inflammation is present; and for muscular weakness and weakness of the sphincter.
- Take 6c/x Nat. Phos. when you have to void frequently and if you have a problem retaining urine. This same cell salt helps with digestive problems that impact on sleep.
- Take 6c/x Kali Phos. for any nonchronic case of incontinence. It helps incontinence problems caused by a nervous condition or state, if urine is hard to retain, or if it is scalding.
- Take 6c/x Nat. Mur., a water-distributing salt, to cut pain after urinating and if there is an involuntary emission of urine while walking. Nat. Mur. plays a vital role in balancing all life processes.

JUMPING OR JERKING LIMBS IN SLEEP

Many adults, especially as they reach an advanced age, can be plagued with an often ignored but difficult problem of periodic leg jerking. It is

Sleep and Restless Leg Syndrome (RLS) and/or Periodic Leg Movement Disorder (PLMD)

Problem	Symptoms	Occurs When/Cause	Effect on Sleep/Other Lifestyle Consequences	Coping Strategies
RESTLESS LEG SYNDROME (RSL)	Unpleasant, creepy, crawly sensations when sitting or lying still, especially at bedtime. • "Feels as if worms are creeping and crawling in my legs." • "Living in hell day and night." • "Sometimes when I am driving or just sitting at the movies or watching TV, I want to keep moving my legs. It drives me crazy."	• Can occur at any age, most severely affected individuals are middle-aged to older. Can first occur during pregnancy. • No known cause, but it often occurs in family clusters. 30% of RLS cases have hereditary cause. Cases that run in families are sometimes more difficult to treat. Scientists searching for RLS gene.	• The continual need to stretch or move the legs to alleviate discomfort and pain interferes with ability to fall asleep. • This leads to extreme tiredness during the day and lack of energy for work or home activities. • Also inability to sit for long periods restricts air and car travel time, participation at concerts, movies, business meetings. All this leads to additional anxiety and depression.	• Home remedies suggested by American Sleep Disorders Association: Some people with RLS respond to the following: hot baths, leg massages, heating pad, ice packs, regular exercise, elimination of coffee. Vitamin E and supplemental calcium have helped some people. • Suggestions from self-help group Restless Legs Syndrome Foundation, Inc.: Tell friends, family and your doctor about your situation.

RESTLESS LEG SYNDROME (RSL) (Continued)

- People with problem often describe symptoms as pulling and gnawing as if they absolutely must move the affected limb. This movement relieves the painful and uncomfortable feelings.

- Other 70% may be connected to poor blood circulation in legs, vitamin or mineral deficiencies, muscle disorders, alcoholism, kidney disease. Other possible triggers: caffeine consumption, smoking, fatigue, too warm in room or prolonged exposure to cold temperatures.

Begin each day with leg stretching exercises. Quick but temporary relief: Soak in a warm bath or take a hot shower. Since sitting for long is a problem, build a desk at counter height. Place computer at counter height. Read while standing up at counter. While walking to offset jumping of legs, listen to books on tape, music or taped lectures. Take aisle and back row seats at movies.

Since legs are less restless in the morning, try to sleep late in early morning hours and/or take afternoon naps. Do not lie in bed to fight RLS. Get out of bed:

- play solitaire, work at your favorite hobby, clean the house.

Sleep and Restless Leg Syndrome (RLS) and/or
Periodic Leg Movement Disorder (PLMD) (continued)

Problem	Symptoms	Occurs When/Cause	Effect on Sleep/Other Lifestyle Consequences	Coping Strategies
PERIODIC LEG MOVEMENT DISORDER (PLMD) Periodic leg movements are not the same as the early night muscle spasms or body jerks (sleep starts) which occur as we fall asleep. These jerks are normal and do not affect ability to sleep or daytime alertness.	Periodic episodes of jerking spells of the limbs during sleeping and sometimes while awake. Movements occur at regular intervals, usually every 30 seconds. Typically, rhythmic extension of the big toe and upward extension of the ankle, knee or hip. Happens usually first half of the night during NREM sleep. Affects about 5% of the population.	Cause unknown. Rare in people under 30 years of age, but more common as people grow older. Men and women equally susceptible. 20% of the people diagnosed with insomnia have PLMD. Common in people who have kidney disease and narcolepsy. Some antidepressant medications may increase the frequency of the limb movements.	Various complaints from difficulty falling asleep, trouble staying asleep or excessive daytime sleepiness. Bed partner may complain of blanket stealing and being kicked. Sufferer may complain that frequent leg movements are wearing the hair off the outside of the legs.	The following good sleep habits are suggested by the American Sleep Disorders Association: • Go to bed at same time every day. • Go to bed sleepy. • Have ritual every night, including warm bath, possibly snack and 10 minutes reading. • Exercise regularly, especially 6 hours before bedtime. Stretch or walk at least 4 hours before bedtime.

PERIODIC LEG
MOVEMENT DIS-
ORDER (PLMD)
(Continued)

- Do not smoke or drink alcohol.
- Nap at same time every day.
- Don't use sleeping pills for more than 3 weeks. Never take sleeping pills after drinking alcohol.
- PLMD is made worse by some anti-depressant medications. Sometimes switching medications may help reduce limb movements.
- If not on an antidepressant medication, investigate herbal aids such as valerian, which comes in capsules, pills and extract.

also known as Periodic Leg Movement Disorder (PLMD) and Restless Legs Syndrome (RLS), which makes their legs and thighs feel creepy and crawly when sitting or lying down. (Such periodic movements are not to be confused with leg cramps.) About 65 percent of adults experience some twitching of the legs (and sometimes the arms) during sleeptime. In mild cases, muscle jerks are infrequent. In strong or severe cases, the unfortunate victim has jerks once or twice a minute. Some people have both problems; they often feel a lot better when they are walking around.

Mild PLMD has very little effect on sleep or daytime alertness. Moderate PLMD brings restless nights, complaints of sleepless nights and a feeling of extreme tiredness during the day. In its most severe form PLMD can be associated with RLS, but, oddly, some people have RLS without PLMD. The overlap is not understood. Sometimes these movements are a precursor to or an indication of the following health problems: anemia, diabetic neuropathy, early kidney disease or venous insufficiency.

COPING STRATEGIES: For normal jumping and jerking in sleep, nutritionists suggest 1000 mg calcium with 500 mg magnesium (always take calcium and magnesium in 2:1 proportion). Restless legs may respond to 400 to 800 IU of vitamin E each day. In *Principles and Practices of Sleep Medicine* Dr. Donald Bliwise says PLMD rarely responds to drug therapy. For alleviation of venous insufficiency he suggests investigating biofeedback of the lower limbs.

TISSUE SALTS (for a thorough discussion of tissue salts see Chapter 8; note that you can buy them in *either* 6c or 6x sizes, which has been abbreviated here as 6c/x):

- Take 6c/x Silica to help with average jerking and twitching of limbs. This tissue salt acts as a cleanser and eliminator while also easing spasms that occur during nighttime.
- Take 6c/x Nat. Sulph. as a specific aid for twitching hands or feet, especially during sleep, or if you wake up tired or sleepy in the morning.
- Take 6c/x Nat. Mur. to help with twitching limbs after a fever. Also use it to restore the body if you feel unrefreshed or tired after a night's sleep.

KIDNEY AND BLADDER INFECTIONS

These infections often interfere with sleep because sufferers have to get up frequently to go to the bathroom.

COPING STRATEGIES: Drink three glasses unsweetened cranberry juice or take cranberry capsules (you can buy both in health food stores). Take goat's milk and only soured dairy products such as yogurt and buttermilk. Take supplements of the following vitamins and minerals: B-complex, B6, C, inositol, choline, acidophilus and calcium and magnesium in a 2:1 ratio.

KIDNEY STONES

Patients with kidney stones have periods of arousal from sleep.

COPING STRATEGIES: Avoid additional urinary tract infections by taking standard cranberry extract in pill or capsule form. Reduce fluid retention with vitamin B6 and counteract antibiotics, which normally destroy good as well as negative bacteria, by adding acidophilus to the daily diet. Count on supplements of vitamin C to acidify the urine and increase internal immune activity; take supplements of magnesium oxide. Taking hot shallow ("sitz") baths is also useful.

MIGRAINE HEADACHES

An aura of flashing bright lights in the form of a vertical zigzag or picket fence (called a "prodrome") precedes most migraines. Nighttime migraines often occur during REM sleep. Migraine patients frequently have difficulties organizing a solid waking and sleeping schedule.

COPING STRATEGIES: Treatment for migraine is most effective if started at the first sign of the aura. Immediately after any warning, take brief, alternating hot and cold showers. Continue the showers as a daily regimen until the headaches pass.

Check into the use of feverfew capsules. In one British study 25 mg of freeze-dried leaves were used successfully in treating migraine victims. In the United States, some naturopathic physicians treat this problem by prescribing up to 1 gram of feverfew.

MENOPAUSE

During menopause, which on average occurs at age 51, women go through a gradual end of their menstrual cycle. During this six-month to ten-year period, women experience a range of physical and emotional changes. While some women sail right through menopause and don't even notice it, many women commonly experience sleep problems, mild to profuse sweating, intense flushes of heat called hot flashes, vaginal dryness and/or occasional mood swings or outbursts of emotions.

During the transition to menopause women tend to have long periods of extremely restless sleep during the night coupled with some daytime sleepiness and a feeling of fatigue. While some women experience bursts of energy (often irritable) after meals, others may have the opposite reaction of sleepiness after eating. Even the calmest women can experience some periods of nervousness, irritability, depression, moodiness and fits of crying. Occasional bouts of forgetfulness can also occur.

STRATEGIES FOR BETTER SLEEP:

- Exercise early in the day. Keep active!
- Eat a number of small, light meals throughout the day instead of three medium ones.
- Don't eat heavy meals at night: allow at least four hours between dinner and sleep.
- If you take ginseng to help with the menopause, take it early in the day to avoid overstimulation near sleeptime.
- If you have hot flashes, don't drink any alcohol, coffee or cola drinks—especially at night. Alcohol and coffee intensify them.
- Experiment with drinking the following before bedtime: warm milk and honey or any of the herbal teas that relax, such as chamomile flowers, hawthorn, hops, lemon verbena or passionflower. (See the section on Herbal Remedies in Chapter 8.)
- If you feel very nervous during the day, take valerian: one 6c/x homeopathic pill, a regular valerian pill or 16 drops of valerian tincture in a tranquilizing herbal tea.
- Take a leisurely hot bath one or two hours before going to sleep. This interval helps create drowsiness as well as a sleep-inducing temperature drop at sleeptime. If you can't take a bath this early in the evening, take one when it's convenient, as it will still help your nightly wind-down. For extra calming action, add these to your bathwater: drops of valerian tincture or a cup of any tranquilizing tea such as catnip or melissa (lemon balm).
- If exhausted before taking a bath, rub your shoulders, chest, arms and knees with apple cider vinegar directly from the bottle. Apple cider vinegar is very restorative. If your skin is delicate or fragile, add eight parts of water to the apple cider vinegar.
- If you wish, alternate apple cider vinegar rubs with invigorating and restorative coarse salt baths: Add a cup of coarse salt to your bath. (See other water therapies in Chapter 9.)
- Make sure your bedroom is quiet and dark. You may wish to use a sleep mask to maintain an even darkness throughout the night.
- See the At-a-Glance Chart in Chapter 4. Remedies include the use of

tissue salts and homeopathic remedies for restless sleep, inability to get to sleep, inability to fall asleep once awakened, if anxious or if the mind won't shut down.

- For sleeplessness during a menopausal period, take 30c/x homeopathic Lachesis every twelve hours for one week.
- For panic attacks that occur in the middle of the night (2 to 3 A.M.), especially because of overwork, take 30c/x homeopathic Calc. Carb. twice a day (every twelve hours) for one week.
- Follow sleep routine habits suggested in Chapter 3, including stopping work at least one hour before bedtime, writing down worries during an "oasis" period, creating a firm going-to-bed time, having massages during the day, turning clocks toward the wall and making sure the room you sleep in is never too hot or too cold.

NUTRITION: Good nutrition and vitamin/mineral supplementation is a key to better health and sleep prior to, during and in the postmenopausal years. To help control hot flashes the following minerals and vitamins are imperative:

- Take calcium and vitamins B5, C and E. The recommended way to take calcium supplements to decrease anxiety and nervousness (and prevent osteoporosis) is to combine it with magnesium in proportions of twice as much calcium as magnesium (2:1 ratio). Vitamins C and E, which increase lagging hormone production, also ease vaginal dryness.
- Take B-complex supplements to enhance the nervous system, and make sure your multivitamin contains zinc.
- Decrease supplements of vitamin A.
- Useful herbs for menopause are small amounts of Ginseng (*Panax ginseng*) and/or Dong Quai (*Angelica sinensis*), both of which contain plant estrogens. Ginseng is a strong general body energizer and stimulant, which increases estrogen production and can decrease periods of depression. Dong Quai is a uterine regulator and tones the entire system during menopause. Other plant estrogens are wild yam (*Dioscorea vilosa*), black cohosh (*Cimicifuga racemosa*) and chaste tree (*Vitex agnus-castus*).
- Menopausal problems are caused by a deficiency of estrogen. So eating plant estrogens in such foods as fennel, parsley, soy and lima beans and a variety of nuts and seeds is extremely useful. Bee pollen (for nonallergic people), dark green vegetables and seaweeds or chlorophyll products can greatly enhance the daily diet and will also help stabilize menopausal symptoms which cause discomfort and influence sleep problems.
- Flaxseed, primrose, black current seed and borage oil, all excellent

sources of essential fatty acids, are exceptionally useful in preventing skin and vaginal dryness and joint stiffness during menopause and can be used prior to menopause to prevent PMS (premenstrual syndrome). The usual dose is two capsules a day. Oil from these capsules, vitamin E capsules or the juice squeezed from an aloe house plant can alleviate the pain of sore breasts if applied externally to the nipples. When taken internally, these same oils, along with profuse amounts of pure water, also can prevent menopausal constipation. To prevent vaginitis and cystitis, add acidophilus capsules or yogurt and freeze-dried cranberry capsules to your daily diet.

EXERCISE AND MENTAL IMAGERY: Stretching, breathing and mind control exercises can greatly influence any discomfort and sleep disturbance that often accompany menopause. (See Chapter 10 for exercises which aid sleep.)

NARCOLEPSY

Narcolepsy is a serious sleep disorder which may involve malfunctioning of sleep regulatory centers. The word comes from the Greek *narké*, for numbness, and *lambanein,* which means "to seize." Narcoleptic people are overpowered with a sudden, uncontrollable attack of sleep. Sometimes there are additional symptoms such as cataplexy (a sudden loss of muscle tension), sleep paralysis and hypnotic hallucinations. During a narcoleptic attack the person goes immediately into the REM dream state. Such irresistible naps can last five to ten minutes or an hour to several hours, and narcoleptics can have eight such naps a day. Attacks are increased in a monotonous or warm environment, after a large meal or after episodes of strong emotions.

Narcolepsy is a life-long disease and the symptoms can increase with aging. The causes are unknown, but there may be a possible involvement with the immune system. Attacks may start because of a head trauma, a central nervous system disease, anesthesia during an operation or because of a family history of narcolepsy. One note of hope: women with narcolepsy sometimes improve during their menopausal years, and sometimes the symptoms disappear entirely.

To solve the problem, the person must first be evaluated by a professional sleep disorders specialist who may be able to control it with medication and close supervision of the patient's blood pressure. Drinking of alcohol must be entirely eliminated. The symptoms of this disorder can improve or worsen spontaneously.

NATURAL REMEDIES: In mild cases, regularly scheduled naps may help avoid attacks. It also helps to achieve optimal fitness, as exercise can sometimes decrease the number of attacks. (See Resources to find out about the American Narcolepsy Association.)

PREGNANCY

Pregnancy can temporarily interfere with restful sleep. During pregnancy, no matter how young the woman is, she has an increasing need to urinate during the night. Some fetuses can be superactive during the night, and their kicking can awaken the mother-to-be. Other common causes for temporary inability to sleep or interruption of sleep are drinking of coffee or use of caffeine products (which may also affect possible birth defects), general overexcitement and worry, nausea and/or heartburn, tension, fatigue, hemorrhoids, leg cramps and sometimes a severe tingling and numbness of the fingers called "carpal tunnel syndrome." During the later months of pregnancy, and most especially during the last weeks, it is often difficult to find a comfortable sleeping position. Irritation of the sciatic nerve, a common problem of pregnancy but one that usually disappears after giving birth, can also interfere with sleep. Even a small deficiency of B-vitamin foods and supplements and an inadequate intake of iron can also cause sleeplessness as well as mood changes.

BEFORE GETTING PREGNANT:

- Make sure your general diet includes all essential nutrients and take a reliable multivitamin/nutritional supplement. Scientists now know that it is imperative to have folic acid in the diet before conception to avoid several birth defects, including spina bifida.
- To avoid excessive urination during the night, build up your pelvic muscle wall by practicing Kegel exercises (tighten the muscles in your vagina and colon as if you were controlling the flow of urine or stopping a stool from emerging). Continue during pregnancy.
- Gradually taper down and eliminate coffee and other caffeine in soft drinks and over-the-counter medications.
- Taper off and gradually eliminate liquor from your diet.

DURING PREGNANCY:

- Establish a regular routine for going to bed. (Read suggestions on safe water therapies, antiworry and dreaming techniques and other relaxation methods in Chapters 9 and 10).
- Avoid stress and fatigue throughout the day; take naps whenever possible.

- Eat as well as possible. Make sure your diet is high in whole grains, green vegetables and other high sources of B-complex vitamins.
- Eliminate all alcohol and caffeine.
- For morning sickness, eat nutritious small meals throughout the day instead of three meals. Keep plain salted crackers by your bedside.
- Ginger may be the pregnant woman's best friend: it's nature's antidote to nausea. Use fresh ginger in cooking, take powdered ginger capsules and don't be stingy with ginger ale, ginger snap cookies or unsugared ginger candy. However, despite the fact of its remarkable abilities, new herbal studies show that pregnant women should not use more than 1 gram of fresh ginger or ginger powder per day.
- Practice yoga deep breathing using your diaphragm all through the day. During episodes of nausea, try the distracting technique of envisioning the most beautiful place you have ever been to. Bring that place to mind as often as necessary, and see yourself happily enjoying this place. Imagine the sounds of the place.
- For heartburn, elevate the head of your bed. Use bromelain enzyme (found in pineapples) capsules to help with digestion.
- To avoid leg cramps, a frequent problem in pregnancy, increase your intake of calcium, potassium and vitamin C. Make sure to include bananas, oranges and grapefruit in your diet every day. Other foods that help control leg cramps are salmon and sardines, soybean products, almonds, sesame seeds and dairy products such as cottage cheese and yogurt (preferably with live acidophilus).

  Stamp your legs on the floor to overcome a cramp. Or apply wet heat by taking a hot shower (end with a short burst of cool water) or using a hot water bottle. Whenever possible when sitting or lying down, elevate your legs so they are higher than your heart. When standing, shift your weight from one foot to the other. Walk as much as possible every day to increase leg circulation.

  Stretch your calves with a "wall pushup." Stand a foot or more away from a doorway with your feet apart and press your upper arms and hands at an angle above you against the doorjamb. Keep your knees straight and feet flat. Repeat with your knees slightly bent, or do one foot at a time.
- Never restrain the urge to urinate. Make sure to void completely in the later months of pregnancy. You can do this by rocking back and forth.
- When going to sleep, use a sleep mask to shut out distracting light.
- Use pillows to comfort and support your body while sleeping on your back and side. While on your back, tuck a rolled towel or a buckwheat eye mask under your neck; lift your knees on a pillow. On your side, use either a long body pillow, now sold through many

mail order catalogs (see Resources), or a series of smaller pillows to tuck under your neck, arms, abdomen and knees.

- The discomfort of carpal tunnel syndrome (CTS), often signaled by extremely painful tingling and pins and needles in the fingers, can occur during pregnancy and disrupt normal sleep. To prevent or control CTS, take three supplements: high doses of calcium/magnesium combinations, vitamin B6 and unsaturated essential fatty acids.
- Avoid repetitive motions with your hands. Do not sleep on your hands or with your hands curled under your head or body. If working at a computer terminal, make sure you are sitting in a supportive chair that is the proper height and distance from the computer. Shake your hands frequently to relax them. Control daytime and nighttime pain by plunging your hands into hot water as often as possible. Massage the neck and shoulder connections to your arms. Have someone else massage those back and shoulder parts you can't reach. In addition, consider TENS (transcutaneous electrical neural stimulator) treatments by a licensed physiotherapist.

TISSUE SALTS AND HOMEOPATHIC REMEDIES: During pregnancy take tissue salts and homeopathic remedies only when absolutely necessary, and never take 3c/x potencies (for a thorough discussion of tissue salts see Chapter 8; note that you can buy them in *either* c or x sizes, which has been abbreviated here as c/x).

CAUTION: DURING PREGNANCY AVOID THE FOLLOWING:
- Apis or combination homeopathic remedies that contain Apis under 30c/x potencies.
- Such herbs as blue cohosh (*Cimicifuga racemosa*), Dong Quai (*Angelica sinensis*), motherwort (*Leonurus cardiaca*) and vervain (*Verbena officinalis*).
- Raspberry leaf tea in the early months of pregnancy, but use it in the last weeks and *especially during labor*. Two other herbs that can *only be used during labor* are Shepherd's purse, which stops bleeding, and wild yam (*Dioscorea villosa*).
- Therapeutic doses of the following herbs: cayenne, cinnamon, fennel or sage. However, they may be used in normal cooking.
- The following uterine stimulants: essential oils of basil (internally or externally), chamomile and celery; celery seeds, wormwood and mugwort (may also cause fetal abnormalities); tinctures of myrrh and goldenseal (internally); and high doses of lavender. However, you can use lavender oil on pillows or dried in sleep pillows.

- Continuous use and/or high doses of ginseng (*Panax ginseng*) and rhubarb root (strong purgative).

SNORING

An estimated 40 percent of the adult population snores. Most snorers suffer some sleep disturbances and sleepiness. "Laugh and the world laughs with you, snore and you snore alone," said Anthony Burgess. Unfortunately, the problem of snoring, like sleep apnea, increases with age and obesity. Snoring, which is caused by partial obstructions of the nasal passages during sleep, creates numerous arousals that cause splintered, irregular sleep each night. This in turn causes daytime sleepiness. Snoring is known to affect heart and circulatory functioning and is identified with hypertension, stroke and some heart diseases. (A more serious snoring disorder—sleep apnea—is described next.)

COPING STRATEGIES: One strategy is to lose weight (which increases snoring) and avoid alcohol and sedatives. Another is not to sleep on your back because it increases snoring. (Special pillows can help you sleep on your side, as sold in the Self Care Catalog in the Resources.)
    Sleep specialists, especially at sleep disorder clinics, can help evaluate

Strategies to Stop Snoring

- Sleep on your side. Some specialists suggest sewing a tennis ball into the back of your pajamas to encourage side sleeping.
- Sleep without a pillow to avoid obstructing airways—unless you use several pillows to completely elevate the head and shoulders.
- Elevate the head of the bed (this also prevents heartburn attacks).
- Do not drink alcohol after 7 P.M., or four hours before bedtime.
- Don't eat big meals at night. Try to eat your largest "dinner" meal at lunch and a lighter lunch at the normal dinner hour.
- Eliminate possible sources of allergy and pollution which may contribute to snoring by installing an air conditioner; putting special filters in the windows; eliminating feather pillows, feather comforters and floor rugs; and exiling all pets from the bedroom.
- Control and reduce excess weight as this strongly contributes to snoring.

the extent of your snoring problem and see if you have sleep apnea. If snoring is not excessive, try any or all of the following self-help devices, including air-cooled steam to ease congestion and help with breathing; any therapeutic steam inhaler; Breathe EZ, a clip that stimulates the septum nerve to open up congested nasal passages; Nozovent, a flexible plastic device that widens the nostrils and helps increase air flow; Snore-No-More, herbal tablets that open the breathing passages (see Resources).

SLEEP APNEA

A special type of snoring, which occurs in at least three million Americans, or about 25 percent of older people, is known as sleep apnea, a medical term for frequent and prolonged episodes when breathing stops during sleep. This continuous pausing in breathing creates low blood oxygen levels, which can cause cardiac arrhythmias, nighttime hypertension, confusion and damage to thinking and functioning. About one in three male snorers and one in five female snorers have sleep apnea. This dangerous type of snoring is really a danger signal, reports Dr. W. Schmidt-Nowara in the August 1995 issue of the journal *Sleep*, published jointly by the American Sleep Disorders Association and Sleep Research Society.

With this condition snoring is very loud and raspy and is followed by a gasp. Often a bed partner reports periods during sleep when the sufferer is not breathing, followed by grunting or snorting sounds as breathing resumes. This pattern of snoring interrupted by pauses, gasps and periods of not breathing continues throughout the night and wakes the sleeper "dozens, even hundreds of times" during the night. The person with sleep apnea has no recollection of any of these awakenings, and even though the snoring is very loud, the patient has absolutely no awareness of snoring or gasping for breath. This type of snoring has many repercussions, including daytime sleepiness, fatigue, impaired thinking upon awakening, recurrent morning headaches, depression and reduced functional capacity. People who have sleep apnea are responsible for five times as many automobile accidents as the rest of the population. Odd sleeping postures are common and the sufferer can fall out of bed or sleepwalk.

COMMON-SENSE MEASURES TO CONTROL SLEEP APNEA (based on material from the American Sleep Disorders Association):
- Get up about the same time every day.
- Go to bed only when sleepy.
- Establish relaxing presleep rituals such as a warm bath, light bedtime snack or ten minutes of reading.

- Exercise regularly, with vigorous exercise in the late afternoon, at least six hours prior to bedtime, and mild exercise, such as simple stretching or walking, at least four hours prior to bedtime
- Keep a regular schedule with set times for eating meals, taking medications and performing chores.
- Avoid caffeine within six hours of bedtime and don't drink alcohol, especially when sleepy. Even a small dose of alcohol when you are tired can have a potent effect. Do not smoke before bedtime.
- Try to nap at the same time every day. Midafternoon is an appropriate time for most people.
- Be very careful about using sleeping pills. Try not to use them at all. Remember that if you have to use them, sleeping pills should never be used for more than three weeks at a time. Never take sleeping pills after drinking alcohol.
- Weight loss is recommended.

Dr. Schmidt-Nowara and her colleagues report that devices called "CPAP" (continuous positive airway pressure) worn in the mouth during sleep reduce and sometimes eliminate snoring. The CPAP keeps the airways open because a low pressure of air is applied through a mask worn over the nose. These devices can be obtained after consultation and evaluation by a sleep disorders specialist.

A SUCCESS STORY: Retired New York State Supreme Court Judge Jerrad Siegal told me of his recent success in combating sleep apnea. He was happy to share his story because professional help from a sleep disorders center completely changed his life.

In many ways the judge's story is quite typical. He didn't know that his snoring was responsible for some of his daytime problems. Judge Siegal recalls, "I had a problem with sleep every night, and of course my wife complained about my loud snoring. During all these years I remember terrible and vivid dreams, dreams in which I was very frustrated. The dreams were so vivid that they were very clear to me the next morning. It was a struggle every morning because I got up enormously tired every day. And the fatigue didn't leave me—I had morning, noon and night fatigue. I was particularly exhausted in the afternoon, and I had to struggle to stay awake. What was really frustrating is that I could only drive my car for a limited amount of time. This really bothered me."

Happily, the judge was sent to Dr. Joyce Walsleben, director of the Sleep Disorders Center at New York University-Bellevue Medical Center, for an evaluation of and solution for his sleep problem. Knocking off weight is the very first treatment for sleep apnea, and he did so. The judge's therapy included the CPAP apparatus, but he disliked it so much he refused to use it. As a compromise his doctor sent the judge to a dentist who specialized in corrective night guards—a mouth bite similar to those used by people who grind their teeth. The dentist designed a night guard to accomplish two things: change the configuration of the judge's mouth and change his bite.

"My mouth guard pulls my jaw over the teeth," explains Judge Siegel, "and this changed my overbite and altered my breathing by pulling my jaw forward." This simple reconstruction and insert has completely changed the judge's life. "I am a new and energetic man now, " says the judge. "I'm never tired. I can drive a car again. I am enjoying life to the utmost. I'm very grateful."

If you have sleep apnea, check with your doctor, and get a referral to a sleep disorders clinic. Many insurance policies cover the costs of crucial consultations, evaluations and devices. You may also want to go to a dentist who specializes in reconstruction of the mouth. Your insurance may also cover the cost of a custom-made mouth bite.

THYROID PROBLEMS

Imbalances of the thyroid show up in two ways: the thyroid can be inactive or overactive. Hypothyroidism (underactive thyroid) manifests itself with sleepiness during the day and lessened ability to do average activities. This medical problem depletes the restorative sleep of stages 3 and 4. Thyroid replacement is necessary, but it is possible to use natural sources. Younger people will quickly bounce back to normal sleep patterns, while elderly people tend to take longer.

Hyperthyroidism (overactive thyroid) brings with it insomnia as well as nervousness and irritability, fatigue, hair and weight loss, sometimes intolerance of heat and protruding eyes. Instead of sleeping 25 percent of the time in stages 3 and 4, people with overactive thyroid have deep sleep states 70 percent of the time. People with overactive thyroid need megadoses of B vitamins and vitamin C along with megadoses of multivitamins, minerals and essential fatty acids to help the glands.

ULCERS

Ulcer symptoms consist of stomach pain, lower back pain, choking sensation, headaches and itching. Ulcers affect sleep because they usually act up in the late evening. The condition increases acid production at night, and this causes discomfort, frequent awakenings and an inability to get back to sleep. The usual drugs prescribed for this problem—Tagamet and

Zantac—sometimes produce a feeling of being unable to fall asleep. The drug cimetidine actually produces insomnia.

COPING STRATEGIES: Many holistic/complementary physicians use standardized licorice pills to inhibit gastric secretions and cayenne pepper capsules to stop the bleeding.

Medications That Can Disrupt Sleep

Ninety percent of the elderly population are on at least one medication, and most are taking at least two medications at the same time. No matter what you take, it's always best to know the correct directions for and the warnings about each medication. Keep in mind that as you age it takes your body longer and longer to metabolize drugs, and the harder it becomes to excrete medicines from the body.

SLEEPING PILLS

Sleeping pills are the most dangerous to take as one gets older, as they remain in the body for a long time and have a cumulative effect. Experts plead with seniors to avoid sleep medications, except perhaps on a temporary basis, since they are only effective for a few weeks and then they cause rebound insomnia. If a doctor is not on the alert for possible repercussions, larger doses are sometimes prescribed. This can cause a dangerous addiction, daytime sedation, confusion, memory loss and impaired driving skills. When withdrawn suddenly, sleeping pills cause a hangover effect, so it's best to taper off gradually. It is especially important to never combine sleep medications with alcohol. Also, avoid sleep medications if pregnant or if you have any liver, kidney or respiratory disease.

BIRTH CONTROL PILLS

A little-known side effect of the hormones in the birth control pill can affect a woman's hormonal balance, which in turn acts on the sleep center. The pills can have a paradoxical effect, and reactions vary. Some women sleep more with the pill; others sleep less than usual. If sleeping too much or too little interferes with a woman's work and home schedule, it's best to check with your physician to readjust the dosage of the pill. (To thoroughly

Taking Medications Can Cause Unwanted Side Effects

The wise medical consumer asks or reads about interactions between two medications. I will never forget having lunch with an attractive, middle-aged friend who, after giving her order, asked if I would remind her later what she had ordered. "I feel so desperate. I seem to have lost most of my short-term memory," she said. I was stunned. I tactfully asked if she was taking any medication, and she said, "Yes, one for sleep and another one for high blood pressure."

Since I know that many drugs do not work well together, but create side effects, I diplomatically suggested that she double-check her medications with her doctor. Surprised and embarrassed, she told me her doctor had been indifferent to her plight. "You are 62—what can you expect from your memory?" he had said. My mouth fell open with indignation, and I persuaded her to contact a new physician. This doctor knew right away that her memory loss was due to the interaction of her two prescription medicines. With a simple change of medication and dosage my friend regained her lost memory! I only hope someday she'll want to try natural remedies for hypertension and sleep.

---

understand the impact of the pill on the body, read Barbara Seaman's classic book *The Doctor's Case Against the Pill*.)

Emotional Problems and Sleep

Life problems such as the grief accompanying the loss of a loved one, financial stresses, retirement, problems with others in ordinary social situations and changes in lifestyle can all cause anxiety and depression. Not having enough to do in the daytime and being bored can also affect sound sleep. Many adults take prescription drugs to combat anxiety and depression, but never connect the drugs with their sleep problems. However, many drugs modify sleep physiology. The side effects vary from innumerable nighttime arousals to desensitization of the nasal passages that either dull or interrupt sleep, a process that can cause or aggravate a preexisting condition of sleep apnea (described above).

Foods That Prevent Sleep

We all know the old folk wisdom: "You are what you eat." This saying is relevant to sleep problems, as the food one eats affects one's health, serenity and ability to hit the pillow and fall asleep instantly. The kinds of foods that have a negative effect on sleep may surprise you.

FOODS HIGH IN SUGAR

Sugar snacks just before bedtime cause a rush in adrenal and endocrine gland activity which interferes with sleep. Eating sugary snacks, in general, while initially giving energy, soon causes an imbalance in blood sugar, which leads to a sudden crash in energy. Eating too much sugar incites the pancreas to emit and escalate insulin delivery. Extra insulin uses needed sugar reserves, causing brain fog and tiredness. The body then uses the adrenal and endocrine glands as if the body were experiencing an emergency, upsetting normal sleep patterns. To improve sleep, eliminate dates, raisins, candies, cookies, cakes, pies and sugared cereals, especially before bedtime.

STARCHES

All starches—corn, potatoes, rice, spaghetti and other flour products—are changed into sugar when digested and then transformed into glucose, which the body uses for energy. However, too much starch can have the same effect as too much sugar. To help promote healthy sleep, eat light carbohydrate meals or snacks at night (see also section entitled "Change Certain Food Habits" in Chapter 3).

BREAD

Always avoid white bread, which is made with white sugar and white flour and has no nutritional value. Eat high-grain bread and then only one slice at each meal. Note that it's nutritionally better to toast whatever bread you eat.

CAFFEINE

Often used to overcome fatigue, caffeine is a strong stimulant which can last in the body from twelve to twenty hours. If ingested late in the day in the form of coffee, tea and cola drinks or hidden in pain killers or other over-the-counter drugs like diet pills, it can interfere with the ability to get to sleep, no matter how tired or sleepy one feels. And this sleep difficulty increases with age. Dr. Peter Hauri of the Mayo Clinic has found that the simple elimination of coffee and other caffeine products from the diet enabled 75 percent of his patients to overcome insomnia.

One cup of coffee may have little effect on sleep, but each additional cup increases the time it takes to get to sleep as well as possible nighttime awakenings and loss of total sleeptime. If one has trouble sleeping, definitely avoid all forms of caffeine late in the day, since caffeine has a stronger impact when taken before sleeptime. Though adults may not be affected by the caffeine in the colas they drink, it just may provoke sleep problems in children. Often the urgent need to urinate both during the day and at night is connected to drinking coffee. Pregnant women and nursing mothers should always avoid caffeine because it may interfere with the healthy growth and development of their children.

As every ardent coffee drinker can attest, suddenly stopping coffee intake creates severe symptoms of withdrawal along with headaches. In fact, many weekend headaches are the result of drinking coffee later in the day than usual during the week. The best way to cut down on coffee is to slowly taper back on consumption. Drink a quarter to a half cup less every day until you reach the reasonable amount of one cup or possibly one and a half cups at breakfast. Women who are trying to get pregnant should immediately start to decrease the amount of coffee to zero before becoming pregnant.

For people who are very sensitive to coffee, try drinking water-decaffeinated coffee or throw away the first cup of tea from a teabag and use the less-strong second emersion. You can always drink herbal table teas such as ginseng, linden, peppermint or vervain. Before bedtime, it's best to drink sleep-provoking herbal teas such as catnip, chamomile and peppermint.

There's one clear indication that caffeine may be the cause of your sleep problems: Do you wake up in the middle of the night unless you've had a cup of coffee before going to sleep? Do you get a strong headache on weekend mornings when you sleep later than usual? Adults who need several strong cups of coffee in the morning or during the day show signs of caffeine withdrawal by getting headaches.

If you think coffee nerves may be the cause of your sleeplessness, try this experiment created by Dr. Hauri. For one week eliminate all caffeine:

"Have no coffee, tea, cocoa, colas, other caffeine drinks, or caffeine medications such as headache pills. If you feel less nervous and tense and sleep better, you may need to eliminate caffeine permanently."

While drinking coffee and taking other caffeine products usually keeps people from sleeping, there are patients with a paradoxical reaction: they get sleepy in the daytime. An article in the *American Journal of Medicine* reported a series of coffee-drinking patients with this condition. Apparently, these patients exhibited a sensitivity to the coffee they had drunk the day before. The assumption of the researchers was that these patients were acting as if they had withdrawal symptoms.

WARNING: Caffeine is included in many over-the-counter and prescription pain pills and cold and allergy pills. Taking two tablets or capsules of these medications several times daily is the equivalent of drinking many cups of coffee. That will certainly interfere with sleep, especially if the medication is taken late in the day. Look for pills that are caffeine-free or are water-based for healing and treating pain. Such natural antipain substances as homeopathic Arnica can be taken internally or used topically as a lotion or ointment.

How Alcohol and Smoking Hinder Sleep

Some people think that having a brandy at bedtime or smoking a cigarette will relax them and make them ready to sleep, but both actually have the opposite effect.

LIQUOR

Drinking alcohol causes fragmented sleep and increases snoring. Not only does it increase the need to urinate, but once the alcohol is absorbed and metabolized, it wakes the drinker up, in contradiction to the sleeper's need. And if frequent urination and sudden arousals weren't enough, the body has the insidious ability of soon tolerating any dose and needing increasingly larger amounts to get drowsy. So if you're drinking to get to sleep—wean yourself—it doesn't work.

If the mere wish to eliminate nightly liquor doesn't work, then investigate the work of the great biochemist Roger Williams. He discovered that the need for alcohol could be overcome with adequate vitamin supplementation, especially with B-complex vitamins and foods. A nutritionist can help you work out a personalized program to overcome this need.

WARNING: When heavy drinkers stop drinking, they may initially have more sleep problems, including many awakenings, increased nervousness, even nightmares. However, sleep disorder specialists report that they can turn these problems around in as little as two weeks.

SMOKING

Because nicotine is a stimulant, smokers have many sleep problems. Heavy smokers can even be awakened by the need to smoke, and once aroused during the night, smokers have a hard time falling asleep again. Moreover, studies have shown that smokers do not get adequate stage 4 restorative deep sleep.

COPING STRATEGIES: Smokenders is an excellent national program that can help you stop smoking for good. (Call the toll-free number 800-828-HELP in the United States to acquire the skills to stop smoking.) The nicotine patch can also be used in conjunction with the program.

Circadian Rhythm Disturbances

If our inborn circadian rhythm is thrown off, for a whole range of reasons, the resulting sleep disturbances can be quite difficult to deal with. Jet lag and doing shift work are common examples. Anyone who has traveled to Europe or Hawaii knows how hard it is to adjust their waking and sleeping pattern to the new time zone and then to readjust back to their usual time schedule once they return home. However, some circadian rhythm disturbances, like advanced- or delayed-phase sleep syndrome and seasonal affective disorder, while less common, are quite devastating. But even these can be successfully treated.

JET LAG UPSETS YOUR SLEEP

According to the National Sleep Foundation, half of all business travelers have a tough time sleeping, particularly on their first night away on a trip. The insomnia that overcomes travelers is often awakening during the night, due to strange new traffic and other street noise, with trouble falling back asleep. Although symptoms usually disappear in about three days, it takes up to a week for the body to adjust to a new time zone. Sleep and light specialists have determined that exposure to sunshine and/or light and

How to Reset Your Internal Clock to Avoid Jet Lag

Prior to Leaving on a Trip

- Purchase the best synthetic melatonin you can obtain, preferably 0.5 mg pills (or cut 1 mg pill in half); be sure it does not contain other substances or additives.
- For a week or more try going to sleep closer and closer to the nighttime of the place where you are going.

FLYING EAST

Day of Departure

On your home time, between 6 and 7 P.M. (if necessary on the flight), take 0.5 mg of melatonin.

On Arrival

- First night at the new time, take 0.5 mg at 9 P.M.
- Take 0.5 mg again at the new bedtime.
- Continue the same dosage for four consecutive nights.
- When taking the dose during these four nights, phase the time down each night by two hours. For example, the first night's dose would be at 9 P.M., the second night at 7 P.M., the third night at 5 P.M. and the fourth day at 3 P.M. Always continue the additional dose at bedtime.

If Flight Continues in Eastward Direction

- If your stay has been less than four days and you plan to continue traveling in an eastward direction: On the day before leaving for the new destination, take 0.5 mg between 6 and 7 P.M. Omit the bedtime dose.
- Day of arrival: Take 0.5 mg at the new local bedtime.
- Continue dosage as above for four nights.

TRAVELING WEST

- Traveling westward is easier on the body and takes a shorter amount of time to recuperate. Sleep researchers say there is little or no advantage in taking melatonin if crossing less than five time zones.

From Europe to New York (Six Time Zones)

- Day before Returning to U.S.: Take 0.5 mg when you wake up in the morning. If you can't take it in the morning, take a dose at bedtime.
- Day of Departure: Take 0.5 mg when you wake up in the morning.
- Arrival at Destination: For four days after you get back, take 0.5 mg at normal home bedtime. If possible, make the timing of the dose later and later each night.

If Stay Is Less Than Four Days and Travel Continues Westward

- Take 0.5 mg at bedtime one night before starting in the westward direction.

---

taking doses of manufactured melatonin can help you fool your body into quickly accepting new time zones.

On recent trips abroad using the method described in the box, I had no jet lag, but rather a seamless, invisible transition into the new time zone. However, the timing of the melatonin must be precise; otherwise you can push your internal clock in the wrong direction. To avoid possible daytime sleepiness, use only short-acting melatonin and no sustained-release products (see Chapter 4 for more about taking melatonin supplements). Note there are different rules for taking melatonin for jet lag depending on whether you're flying east or west.

Some people have permanent jet lag, which is another type of adult circadian rhythm disturbance. People with this problem can't seem to fall asleep at the "right" time—ever. Their body is out of synchronization with the world they live in. These people fall asleep at a completely different time each day, which has a disastrous effect on work and home schedules. Victims of this internal clock upset can be quickly and easily helped by sleep disorder specialists. Step-by-step reprogramming techniques can also be used.

Given Hilton Hotels interest in the welfare of their many business travelers, they have established sleep-tight rooms, on a limited basis, in certain key U.S. cities. Here visitors can experiment with sound devices that duplicate a rainfall or a soothing fan, use breathing and relaxation tapes or try "circadian light boxes" that help reset jet-lagged body clocks. Why not take a cue from this hotel chain and carry the following in your flight bag: a specific schedule of melatonin use (see box), a sleep mask, ear plugs (nonswimming) and a portable tape machine with breathing, relaxing and sound-sleep-inducing tapes. Frequent fliers can also purchase visor-light devices that carry instructions on resetting one's internal clock.

SHIFT WORKERS

The decline in productivity is greatest among shift workers since they repeatedly must work when their body clock feels sleepy. It is estimated that 80 percent of shift workers—including pilots, railroad and subway engineers, air control dispatchers, cab drivers, factory workers, firemen and police officers, business travelers and diplomats—all have trouble sleeping because their work puts them at odds with their own internal biological clock. In 1991 the federal government reported that one in five full-time workers, or almost 15 million people, worked nonstandard hours that year. Each day since then thousands of American and transnational firms have expanded their global operations and put their workforce on 24-hour schedules. Commonly those who work nonstandard hours work at night or rotate 8-hour shifts around the clock. Elsewhere in the industrial world 20 percent of workers are on rotating night and early morning shift.

Workers who put in long hours during the night or who rotate through different work schedules are often sleep-starved because they are obliged to go against their own biological alertness and sleep clocks. The body is naturally geared to be more alert in the morning and early evening, with a modest dip in the early afternoon. Energy plunges between midnight and sunrise. Consequently, shift workers on the whole get one hour less sleep a day than other workers on a steady daytime schedule. It is important to recognize that the body repairs itself with adequate sleep and that sleep is essential to accomplish routine mind or physical tasks with ease and clarity.

A Swedish study supported by the Swedish Work Environment Fund and the Swedish Medical Research Council says that it seems sensible for "night workers to prevent some of the night shift fatigue by taking an afternoon (or evening) nap. This is of increasing importance the more vigilance is required to carry out the tasks."

The report suggests that each shift worker try out naps at different times and of different lengths of time to note the optimal effect. Should there be a problem in creating a nap schedule, it helps to reduce the time of sleep during the day after the night shift. The study concludes, "This suggestion may seem strange, since it would cause a sleep deficit. However, if this procedure helps to initiate and maintain an afternoon nap, the net effect would presumably be to lessen night-shift fatigue."

There are many things shift workers can do to help themselves:

- Create an inviting, safe, comfortable and quiet place to sleep. Try to sleep long enough to get up feeling rested.
- Establish a realistic and protective sleep routine (see Chapter 3).

- Expose yourself to early morning light—either daylight or bright artificial light.
- Take planned naps. For instance, the FAA (Federal Aviation Administration) now permits pilots on long hauls to take scheduled naps while the co-pilot controls the airplane because it's been shown that this increases pilot alertness.
- Sleep experts suggest that the average shift should only last three weeks.
- To conform to your own biological clock, request that your shifts move clockwise or forward. That means starting the first shift in the earlier part of the day and going forward towards evening, then nighttime. It's best not to move shifts back and forth or backwards.
- When shift work brings on insomnia, it is possible to reset one's biological clock with timed exposure to bright artificial light. This can be accomplished by utilizing a sleep disorders specialist (many companies can bring specialists in to work with a large group of workers) or sometimes by your own personal investigation of light therapy. Lights that help with sleep and winter depression are listed in the Resources.
- Check the information on resetting one's biological clock with behavior modification sequences (described below) and judicious use of melatonin supplementation (Chapter 4).

ADVANCED- OR DELAYED-PHASE SLEEP SYNDROME

Children and adults, especially as they get older, can get out of sync and have problems with normal getting-up and going-to-sleep patterns. To understand the concept of an advanced or delayed internal clock, it might help to visualize a grandfather clock with a huge pendulum. If the pendulum advances too fast or slows down too much, it must be adjusted. The same is true of our body clock. When the internal clock gets out of sync and advances,impels people to go to sleep much too early. This is called advanced-phase sleep syndrome. Sometimes this also causes a problem in falling back to sleep if aroused during the night. When the internal clock is delayed, it obliges the person to go to sleep very late. This is called delayed-phase sleep syndrome. This problem also causes that droopy, sluggish, languid, depressed feeling that so many people get at the height of the winter months.

Advanced-phase sleep syndrome is best described by an Indiana friend who was distressed by the sleep habits of her husband. "I feel as if I am living on the East Coast, he is living on the Pacific Coast, and never the twain shall meet. It's like I'm living alone because we have to eat dinner no later than 5 P.M. since he has to be in bed by 8 P.M. Poor guy, he

Bedtime Reconditioning

Sleep researcher Dr. Elliot Phillips devised the following drastic ten-day, no-nap body rescheduling and bedtime reconditioning for people whose time clock is completely off. It's ideal for insomniacs who go to bed too late enight and get up far too late each morning. The process involves reshaping one's timetable in order to reset the body clock to a better wake-and-sleep sequence.

Each day for ten days the person goes to bed several hours later than usual each night and wakes up several hours later in the morning. During the ten days the body is totally baffled by the experience. The reconditioning works eventually because one circles the clock until one arrives at the wakeup and sleeptime needed for daily life. Some people must do this clock rotation twice before it finally works.

TIMETABLE	GO TO BED	GET OUT OF BED
First Night	5 A.M.	1 P.M.
Second Night	7 A.M.	3 P.M.
Third Night	9 A.M.	5 P.M.
Fourth Night	11 A.M.	7 P.M.
Fifth Night	1 P.M.	9 P.M.
Sixth Night	3 P.M.	11 P.M.
Seventh Night	5 P.M.	1 A.M.
Eighth Night	7 P.M.	3 A.M.
Ninth Night	9 P.M.	5 A.M.
Tenth Night	Anytime after 9 P.M.	No matter what time you go to bed, get up at the time you have decided you should always get up each morning.

can't ever sleep straight through and gets up to urinate all through the night. And by 3 A.M.—when I am fast asleep—he is getting up and out. But because he gets up all through the night, he gets infernally tired all through the day, and just when I want to go shopping or share something with him, he is off to a long nap. It is driving me crazy! We never can do anything together anymore, and we can't do any socializing at night." This typical advanced-phase circadian rhythm disturbance happens a lot to very elderly people. Only this Indiana man was young—in his early sixties! His problem, as well as the opposite, delayed-phase syndrome (where one doesn't sleep at night, but sleeps during the day), both respond to slow changes in the sleep schedule (see box on bedtime reconditioning) and to the use of a judiciously low dose (0.5 mg) of melatonin, in addition to timed light therapy (described below).

REDUCED DAYLIGHT IN WINTER CAN CREATE SLEEP PROBLEMS: SEASONAL AFFECTIVE DISORDER

Everyone who lives in a northern climate knows how many things can go by the boards in the cold, short days of winter. Experts have determined that at least 25 percent of the population in the middle to northern latitudes have winter blahs. The reaction to these shortened hours of daylight varies from person to person. For instance, until I did my own light therapy, I always went into winter doldrums by the end of January and all February. Unless I get into the sun, do a lot of physical exercise at the gym or have an extremely demanding project I'm concentrating on, I get logy, lethargic and tend to crave sweets and carbohydrates.

When people are especially sensitive to shortened daylight, the winter blues, known as "Seasonal Affective Disorder" (SAD), generally cause one or more depressive symptoms. Common symptoms include the need to sleep more, sometimes as much as four extra hours a day, or, paradoxically, the inability to fall asleep or sometimes sleeping less; increased appetite, especially for sweets and carbohydrates; heightening of menstrual problems; the need to be more solitary and less social; a despondent feeling of not being able to cope at the job and a lassitude about doing home chores; exhaustion, fatigue and generalized depression.

Because pioneer sleep researchers found that melatonin was only manufactured in darkness, they reasoned that light could be used to restore certain sleep functions. Through research it was discovered that average light intensity from a reading lamp had no effect on human melatonin production, but when multiplied five times, the light had a profound effect. These intensified amounts, measured in lux units, could overcome SAD and shift work irregularities. Light works on an opposite curve to melatonin. Therefore morning light and late afternoon melatonin can be used separately and as a complementary and cohesive (timed) twofold therapy to achieve desired results.

Bright Light Therapy

About fifteen years ago, Dr. Alfred Lewy of the Sleep Disorders Research Section at Oregon Health Sciences University in Portland had a patient who asked for help with his recurrent wintertime depression (SAD). Since the internal body clock is very sensitive to bright light and darkness, Dr. Lewy took this opportunity to research whether the man would respond to bright light therapy. Within three days of light therapy, the patient and the nurses controlling the case saw a big change in the man—and chronobiological and mood disorders light therapy was born!

Winter depression is generally considered a delayed-phase sleep syndrome, which is why morning light given between 6 and 9 A.M. is used to treat the problem. Morning light advances the clock and helps you get up earlier. People usually see a noticeable improvement in mood within four to five days, although some patients can take several weeks to show a positive response.

Light therapy involves sitting under intense bright light—five times stronger than regular house lights—for a specific time of day and for certain lengths of time. The effect changes the shorter winter day into a longer spring day of 13 1/2 hours. The level of light duplicates the intensity of light provided outdoors at either sunrise or sunset. (Specifications for different lighting systems vary since they deliver different amounts of light.) The only caution about using real sunlight is to remember not to look directly at the sun, as it can harm the eyes.

Dr. Norman E. Rosenthal, chief of Environmental Psychiatry at the National Institutes of Mental Health, reports how researchers treated sleep problems of SAD patients with a bedside lamp connected to a second light source programmed to create an artificial dawn. "They found the simulated dawn to have antidepressant effects," reports Rosenthal in JAMA (12/8/93), "even though the patients were asleep while being treated, and the final intensity (250 lux) was considerably lower than that required by conventional light therapy." Rosenthal mentions that while SAD "occurs most commonly as a result of the short, dark days of winter, [it] may also be due to dark indoor working environments, unseasonable cloudy spells, or ocular difficulties."

Side Effects

The side effects of light therapy are minimal, if any. In the beginning of treatment, a few people do react to the intense lights, possibly with a feeling of unease, others with slight nausea. One effect—increased dryness in the eyes—can be overcome with artificial liquid tears and/or a home humidifier. To avoid possible bacterial contamination, always clean the humidifier out every day. According to Dr. Rosenthal, "While light therapy is often free of side effects, the more common ones include headaches, eyestrain, irritability, and insomnia, the last particularly if treatments are administered late at night. . . . When side effects occur, they are almost always mild and can generally be handled by decreasing the duration of treatments or by having the patient sit a little farther from the light source."

Cautions in Use

Light therapy should be carefully supervised by your ophthalmologist if you have retinitis pigmentosa, diabetic retinopathy or macular degeneration.

If you suffer from SAD, you may need intense light therapy. So take a light check:

- Are you working in a dark indoor environment?
- Are the rooms in your living quarters dark or dim?
- Are your reading lights small and inconvenient?
- Are overhead lights set high or with nonbright shades?
- How is the light in the kitchen?
- How is the light where you eat your dinner?

Lighten your winter moods by replacing reading, desk and kitchen lamps with full-spectrum bulbs (see Resources). I've been using full-spectrum bulbs throughout the year for the last several years, and they have greatly decreased my winter doldrums.

If you suffer from major winter depression, you can take more extreme measures:

- Buy fluorescent bulbs at least five times stronger (measured in lux units) than ordinary light bulbs, and install them in a box with a diffusing screen.
- Sit near the lights with your eyes open, turn your body and head in the direction of the lights, but do not look directly at the lights. Reading and eating are good activities during this time.

- Treatment time varies, lasting fifteen minutes or longer. It is critical to stay within guidelines recommended by your physician or the light mechanism manufacturer on how far to sit from the light and how long the treatment should last. (One new light mechanism fits on the head like a cap and allows you to do all your home chores as you move around. See Resources.)
- Researchers have found it is best to begin treatment as early as the fall and continue throughout the winter into spring. In the spring outdoor light is usually enough to restore high energy and mood once again.
- Don't skip treatment days. Research proves that even a three-day lapse in treatment can cause a setback in mood, energy and appetite.

(See Resources for a listing of the Society for Light Treatment and Biological Rhythms.)

3

Positive Sleep Strategies

One thing unites all insomniacs. Each anticipates trouble falling asleep or getting back to sleep when aroused during the night. Problem sleepers can conquer their sleep resistance if they devise and live by a comfortable and pleasant nightly routine. The routine works in two ways. It instructs the brain to expect an orderly (circadian) sleep-wake rhythm. And, of equal importance, it replaces the fear of not being able to get to sleep or, if aroused, to fall asleep again, with an expectation of sleep.

When patients in sleep labs are deprived of any light or time cues, something interesting happens: the day is no longer 24 hours, but becomes a 25-hour or longer day. Sleep researchers have noted that these patients appear to need a natural nap between 2 and 4 P.M. If you are sleep deprived and find you must nap, try a brief ten-to fifteen-minute snooze close to 2 P.M. Many high-achieving, famous men of the past and present nap each day. One such was the late film producer Harry Warner of Warner Brothers Studio, who was in the habit of taking an afternoon nap in his office. It was an unwritten rule of the studio that he was not to be disturbed. On one occasion, however, film star Bette Davis burst into the office while Warner was asleep and began ranting about a script that did not meet with her approval. Without opening his eyes, Warner reached for the phone and called his secretary. "Come in and wake me up," he said. "I'm having a nightmare." Miss Davis could not help laughing, and the crisis over the script was resolved in a few minutes.

Habits That Help You Sleep

Many habits can be changed or new ones adopted that will help you sleep better and feel more rested and refreshed after you sleep, especially the following.

ANYONE CAN BENEFIT FROM A NAP

Winston Churchill was a famed instant sleeper. In *Of Men and Plants* he tells Maurice Messegue, "I told you, I'm as healthy as a baby. Have you ever noticed how all babies look like me? And d'you know why I look so rested? Because I can drop off to sleep anywhere at any time."

However, there is controversy about whether a person with insomnia should ever take a nap, especially since a nap at the wrong time of day can put an entire sleep schedule into jeopardy. However, most sleep experts agree that naps are an excellent method of catching up on lost sleep. Taking a short ten- to thirty-minute nap during a lunch break or as near to 2 P.M. as possible will provide a sleep-deprived person with more satisfied rest than any extra time appended to the morning wakeup time.

Naps can really be helpful if you're planning an active night; catching a refreshing nap in the afternoon will work wonders. If you are at home during the day and know that your nighttime activities will demand alertness and energy:

- Take a long, hot bath. Use the friction and salt rub techniques described in Chapter 9. Get into bed wrapped in your towel under warm bedclothes.
- Darken the room as much as possible. Wear a sleep mask to intensify the feeling of darkness.
- To make sure you awaken on time, tell yourself you want to sleep about a half an hour. Your own body clock should wake you up. If you aren't sure you can do this, set the alarm for half an hour.

CREATE A WORRY-TIME OASIS

Sometime after dinner, for five to ten minutes, sit down in a quiet corner away from everyone else, and with a pad and pencil, scribble whatever comes to mind about anything that is bothering you. If solutions or schedules of action come to mind, write them down. This unremarkable daily act will clear internal brain static from your sleeping mind: small or sometimes long-range concerns, financial worries, details of future projects, ruminations about a perplexing or upsetting incident or personal interactions. As soon as you expose these concerns and write them down, solutions tend to crop up, worries are lifted and anxieties should not thrust themselves into your nighttime falling-asleep routine.

If, despite writing a worry-time list, you can't shake one particular idea, a remarkable Bach flower remedy banishes tenacious ideas. All you need is a few drops of White Chestnut under the tongue.

A 150-Year-Old Antiworry Technique

One day, President Abraham Lincoln's Secretary of War, Edwin Stanton, came to him with a strong complaint about an officer who had disobeyed or failed to understand an order. "I think I'm going to sit down, write a letter and give that officer a strong piece of my mind," said the Secretary.

"Do so," nodded Lincoln. "Write him now while you have it on your mind. Make it sharp. Cut him all up." Stanton was astonished that Lincoln gave him such an unqualified go-ahead, and he quickly wrote the angry letter. He asked permission to return to the Oval Office and read his powerful letter to the President.

"Why, that's a good letter!" said Lincoln encouragingly.

Stanton was pleased at Lincoln's approval. "How shall I send it on to the front?" he asked.

"Send it?" said Lincoln. "Why, don't send it at all! Tear it up! You have freed your mind on the subject, and that is all that is necessary. You never want to send such letters; I never do. Before I go to bed, I write a list of all the important things on my mind—that frees my mind of worries and I sleep a lot better for it."

ADJUST YOUR INTERNAL BIOLOGICAL CLOCK WITH LIGHT

If you usually have trouble getting to sleep, take an early morning walk in sunlight, or if you live in a sunless climate, expose yourself, particularly your eyes, to strong artificial light. Light in the morning tells the pineal gland to emit melatonin, the sleep/wake hormone, early in the evening so that you feel sleepy when you go to bed. Conversely, if you are going to sleep much too early, try the technique of delaying your internal biological clock by standing or walking in sunlight or strong artificial light in the late afternoon or early evening.

CHANGE CERTAIN FOOD HABITS

- Avoid heavy, late meals before bedtime: Eating late at night interferes with solid sleep. To make sure you stay alert during the day, always have some protein for breakfast and lunch. Carbohydrate meals are good at night because they help introduce tryptophan, the precursor to serotonin, which in turn is the precursor to melatonin, the sleep/wake hormone.
- However, some people need a nighttime snack: Years ago a friend astonished me by complaining she was impelled to get up every night—in the middle of the night—to nibble on cookies or cake. I wondered about her seemingly strange habit. Now I know she was one of many people who have a deep drop in blood sugar at night, a problem called "nighttime hypoglycemia." The problem is easily rectified by eating a small, high carbohydrate snack just before going to sleep. It also helps to sip on sedative herbal tea.

AVOID LIQUIDS TO STOP URINATING DURING THE NIGHT

If you want to avoid getting up at night to urinate, try to drink most of your necessary eight glasses of pure water early in the day. Also, except for certain soporific herbal teas, cut back on all other liquids after three or four o'clock in the afternoon. Caffeine is a noted interrupter of sound sleep. A morning cup of coffee is all right for most people, but remember that caffeine stays in the system from 10 to 20 hours! Avoid drinking coffee and any caffeinated soft drinks or taking over-the-counter medicines after 12 noon.

Another liquid that creates a lot of sleep problems is liquor. Dr. John Navard, secretary of the British Medical Association, said in a speech, "Alcohol is the most powerful depressant of the central nervous system available in this country without a doctor's prescription. If it were being introduced now it would be a controlled drug." Millions of people who want to avoid sleeping pills assume they are safe imbibing a small nightcap to get to sleep. Most of these people don't realize that some of their fragmented sleep is the result of that nightcap. As soon as the alcohol is metabolized, it no longer allows you to sleep, but acts to arouse you. This habit can also cause small or full-blown depressions. It is especially important never to drink alcohol if you are taking sleeping pills.

GO TO BED AT A REGULAR TIME

Even if your personality resists a strict routine and if you are an insomniac, this is one realm in which you need to have an I-have-to-do-it-even-if-it-doesn't-feel-natural attitude. First, figure out what time of the day you need to wake up for work or other activities. Or if you are going to bed much too early every day, what hours of the evening would you like to be awake to have a more normal social life? Then plan on going to bed and arising to fit in with your work and social needs. Also, add some personalized details to your bedtime routine—small signals that sleeptime is coming up. These can be as simple as taking a warm bath and toweling yourself dry in a specific way, repeating a melodious fragment of your favorite poetry or sounding out a yoga mantra such as OHM MANE PADNE OHM over and over. Something as innocuous as fluffing your bed pillows a certain way just as you are going to sleep may also help.

Janice Huggins of San Diego uses this time for what she calls "body validation." She closes her eyes and mentally goes over her entire body from head to toe. When she finds an area that hurts or feels stiff, she breathes deeply and mentally sends her breath to that area. Then she stretches and massages the stiffness.

Plan your own routine and rituals to reinforce your sleep mode. Thereafter, within reason, no matter how fascinating you find a TV movie or a chat on the phone with a friend, go to sleep at the same time each night and get up at the same time each morning, even on weekends. The weekend stricture is important, because without consistency every day the routine falls apart. It is often hard to dispense with old habits and approaches to sleep. That famous insomniac Mark Twain admitted a habit could not just be tossed out a window. Said Twain, "It must be coaxed down the stairs a step at a time."

TAKE A RELAXING BATH EACH NIGHT

Hot or warm water soothes the skin and relaxes the mind and the body, while vigorous toweling promotes fresh circulation of the blood. If you take the bath two hours before climbing into bed, it has the added advantage of creating a valuable sleep-provoking drop in temperature at just the right time for sleep. (Also consult Chapter 9 for other water therapy.)

CULTIVATE HELPFUL BED HABITS

- Make your bed a comfort-free zone: Make sure you only use your bed for sleeping and making love. Don't read, don't eat and don't watch television in your bed. Make sure your bed is comfortable and firm. If you do have any allergies such as to feather pillows or other feather products, be sure to eliminate them from your bedroom. Down pillows are soft but can lead to allergies.

  Dust mites are a danger in the bedroom, on the bed itself and on the pillows, blankets or comforters. First, eliminate any possible allergy provokers, then wash all your pillows and cover each pillow in not one but two zippered pillowcases. (To obtain totally nonallergic bedding, consult the Resources.)
- Are you sharing a bed with a blanket hog or snorer?: Temporarily move into another room until you can establish a new, sounder sleep schedule. Some strong snorers have a condition called "sleep apnea" (see Chapter 2), which can be overcome with a variety of breathing apparatus obtainable from sleep disorder specialists at hospital centers.
- Two bed pillows support the knees and alleviate severe back pain: Since I have a knee injury, I find the very best way to start my night of sleep is to use two pillows, which equal the height of my thigh, to lift my legs. I don't start out with any pillow under my head, but just lift my knees and my legs onto the larger pillows. I relax this way for about ten minutes, toss the knee pillows out of the bed, grab two other small pillows to clutch and lie on and begin the serious effort of going to sleep.

  Incidentally, the above position also alleviates severe back pain. If you go to sleep with back pain and wish to lie this way most of the night, make sure the height of the pillows is about the height of your thighs. Do not put a pillow under your head, but support any accidental roll or shift with two small pillows on either side of the head.
- Wear loose, comfortable nightclothes: Wear warm clothes in the winter and cool clothes in the summertime.
- Turn your alarm clock to the wall: You will sleep much better if you are not checking up on yourself during the night and fretting about time lost being awake.

SLEEP AT THE PROPER TEMPERATURE

"Neither a borrower nor a lender be," Polonious instructs his son in Shakespeare's *Hamlet*. If sleep research had been available in the 16th century,

Shakespeare would have added, "Be neither too hot nor too cold when you go to sleep."

One night a sore throat forced me to ignore this dictum. In addition to several other natural nostrums, I tried to keep my throat warm with a silk turtleneck blouse. I didn't realize how hot that would keep my arms and chest, so I tossed and turned, too hot to fall asleep. Finally about 2 A.M., I whisked off the turtleneck and the cool air made my temperature drop. I fell asleep instantly.

Even if you live in a terribly cold climate and have to go to bed with socks on, as soon as your body is warm, take off the socks. Despite the fact that down covers can cause allergies for some, I'm a strong advocate of cotton-covered down because it allows the body to be heated in a natural fashion. With a proper down cover, you are rarely too hot nor can you be cold.

What about electric blankets? Avoid them for two reasons: While they elevate the temperature, they do not allow the body to lower its temperature, which it must normally do to fall asleep. Further, many electromagnetic researchers feel electric currents may be implicated in breaking our defenses against cancer. When you need a way to get warm fast, take a hot bath and get into bed instantly. With a reliable blanket or down cover, you will be able to maintain natural, normal and proper heat.

SLEEP IN THE DARK

The sooner the room is absolutely dark, the quicker your pineal gland will secrete normal amounts of the sleep/wake hormone melatonin, which is only manufactured in darkness. That is one of the reasons why insomniacs find wearing a dark sleep mask to keep out stray light is an invaluable sleep aid.

Also, try a Japanese-style silk-encased rice or buckwheat eye pillow prior to putting on the mask. Perhaps it is the silk or it may be the delicate weight, but these pillows give indescribable comfort to tired eyes. Once in a while, for added comfort, squeeze an eye pillow under your sleep mask.

CREATE SOUND BARRIERS

Some people are very sensitive to loud sounds, and as we grow older, noise can become a hidden stress. Overcome noise sensitivity by sleeping in a quieter spot in the house or adding thick, dark curtains to draw during the night.

Many noise-sensitive people find solace in ear plugs or ear muffs while they sleep. One dependable brand used in noisy factories and found in most drugstores is called Noise Filter (see Resources). Do not use ear plugs that are designed for swimming because they don't eliminate sound. You can cover outside or household noises with the neutral "white sound" from a fan, air conditioner, a white noise machine or cassettes that play the hypnotic sounds of the ocean or a summer country night in a garden. If household noises tend to awaken you too early, put foam mats under appliances in the kitchen. Protect against noise stress by taking additional B complex and vitamin C supplements.

TELL YOURSELF THAT YOU ARE GOING TO SLEEP

You will wonder how you ever lived without this concept, for it is as simple as stating your intention of going to sleep quickly and soundly. As you lie down, tell yourself something like this: "I will sleep instantly, and tomorrow I'll get up at 7:15 and feel great and refreshed. Immediately after breakfast, I'll go to work and. . . ." If this doesn't work instantly, try one or several of the physical exercises in Chapter 10.

CHILDHOOD MEMORIES HELP BREAK INSOMNIA

Sometimes all it takes to break a long period of sleeplessness is to recall a happy sleep routine from childhood. How good it was to be loved and tucked in. How safe it felt. How wonderful it was to have no cares and to sleep "like a baby." Many adult insomniacs have overcome their problems by remembering what it was like to be a young kid.

COPING WITH NIGHTTIME AWAKENINGS

From birth on, it is normal to be awakened during sleep. It is also normal not to remember the arousals and go right back to sleep.

Some sleep scientists think these awakenings may be part of our prehistoric heritage when it was important to check and recheck one's safety. Teenagers are aroused from sleep about five or six times a night, while young and slightly older adults are aroused more often. No one knows why, but many elderly people may wake up as often as one hundred times during each night's sleep.

COPING STRATEGIES: There is no need to be alarmed about the arousals; the idea is to train yourself to cope with them by using one or more of the safe, natural approaches presented here.

- If you cannot get back to sleep within ten to fifteen minutes, do not linger in bed and brood about how hard it is to get back to sleep.
- Get out of bed and walk around briefly.
- Do not turn on the TV! (It's too tempting and overstimulating.)
- If you're still awake after a brief walk, sit down and do something boring: read a dull book, play several games of solitaire or polish shoes, brass or silver. Knitting is excellent. All these produce eye fatigue. If I'm ever at a point when my normal imagination exercises haven't worked, I get out of bed and play solitaire on my computer, or I embroider a fragment for one of my "stained glass" crazy quilts.
- Consider just sitting in the dark and listening either to music or to parts of a book on tape.

DEALING WITH "SUNDAY-NIGHT INSOMNIA"

Some people suffer from an end-of-the-weekend insomnia induced by thinking about future chores and next week's problems. Dr. Thomas Roth, director of the Sleep Disorders and Research Center at the Henry Ford Hospital in Detroit, says, "The challenge in overcoming this type of insomnia is that after a while our bodies become conditioned to react in this way: that is, our expectation of sleeplessness becomes as much a contributing factor to the problem as the worry itself." Dr. Roth reports that this conditioning can turn occasional insomnia into chronic insomnia, and he urges patients to do something about it as soon as possible. In addition to advising these patients to avoid work-related activities in the bedroom, he helps them relieve anxiety by preparing in advance as much as possible for the next morning:

- Pick out clothes for the next day.
- Pack your briefcase.
- Rehearse your presentation (or whatever is needed for the next day's success).

Summary of Key Points to Overcoming Insomnia

- Personalized routines create an expectation of sleep and reinforce brain patterns that regulate one's circadian rhythm.
- Keep to the same rhythmic routine, going to bed and getting up in the morning time, even on weekends.
- If you can't get to sleep easily at night, walk in sunlight in the morning. If you go to bed too early every night, walk in sunlight in the afternoon.
- Several hours before bedtime, jot down worries on a pad.
- Don't eat late or heavy meals. Nighttime hypoglycemics should eat a light carbohydrate snack just before going to bed.
- Drink needed water early in the day, and in general decrease fluid intake after the noonhour.
- Avoid rebound insomnia by eliminating nightcaps of liquor.
- To avoid being awakened by outside light, wear a sleep mask.
- Create sound barriers in your room, and use your own version of hypnotic white noise to lull you to sleep.
- Make sure your bed is firm and nonallergenic.
- Avoid sleeping pills, especially as you age. They take a long time to get out of the system and can cause serious medical problems as well as deeper, boomerang insomnia.
- Calcium pills before bedtime release tryptophan, the precursor to melatonin, to the brain. You can now get tryptophan by prescription from a physician.
- The clock is an enemy of the insomniac. Just as you are going to bed, turn it to the wall so you can't see it glaring during the night.
- Induce sleep by reducing temperature with a relaxing bath every night.
- Last thing before getting into bed, visit the bathroom.
- Take a few minutes to establish a constructive dreaming routine. Just before going to sleep, jot down one sentence summarizing one problem you need to solve. Allow your dreaming mind to solve it while you sleep (see Chapter 10).
- Recapture carefree childhood sleep by recalling the best things about going to sleep when you were a child.
- If awakened and can't get back to sleep, don't brood; get out of bed and do a boring task before returning to sleep again.

Foods That Promote Sleep

Fortunately, the diet that protects against chronic diseases such as cancer, heart attack, diabetes and high blood pressure is also the right diet for people with sleep problems. Fresh foods are best as an initial source of vitamins and minerals, but often toxic elements in the environment—air, water and pesticides found on foods—interfere with total absorption. So choose your foods wisely and well. A thorough study of the nutritional elements found in various foods is highly recommended for optimal health.

Certain foods produce the amino acid called "tryptophan" that will help you get to sleep. For foods that contain high amounts of tryptophan, try warm milk or small amounts of turkey, tuna fish or cheese.

SALADS AND FRESH VEGETABLES

Eat fresh greens, fruits and vegetables throughout the day, especially at lunch and supper, and including breakfast, when possible.

Salads and fresh vegetables have a positive effect on sleep because they are easy to digest and are a wise choice with chicken and fish or vegetable protein for a dinner meal. Protein helps prevent hunger pangs during the night. It's best to avoid heavy meals for dinner, as they are difficult to digest and may keep you awake during the night. Reserve lunch for the big meal of the day.

WHOLE GRAINS AND FIBER FOODS

Eat one slice of whole fiber bread at each meal. Complex carbohydrates from whole grains, along with vegetables, fruit, potatoes and salads, can reduce the risk of certain cancers, high blood pressure, heart disease and diabetes. Whole grains and fibers also are instrumental in lowering cholesterol and triglycerides.

Vitamin and Mineral Supplements That Aid Sleep

Supplements of vitamins and minerals can be an enormous help in staving off disease, feeling tip-top and achieving adequate sleep. Often it helps to use time-release supplements, unless otherwise noted. Plan on taking them several times a day after meals.

CALCIUM

Calcium is essential for the nervous system, and a minor deficiency often causes insomnia. Calcium releases the amino acid tryptophan which helps the body manufacture the sleep/wake hormone melatonin. This natural sedative is important in preventing muscle cramps, a known sleep inter-rupter. We often lose calcium because of stress and tension which pour large amounts of lactic acid into the bloodstream, making assimilation of calcium impossible. So despite eating large amounts of foods rich in cal-cium, such as dairy products and green, leafy vegetables, the body can actually crave calcium.

Calcium works with magnesium and should always be in a 2:1 propor-tion: two times calcium to one of magnesium. Calcium citrate is said to be the most easily absorbed of the supplements. The recommended dose of calcium, especially for someone with sleep problems, ranges from 800 mg for adults to 1200 mg for teenagers, pregnant women, nursing mothers and menopausal women. It's best to time small doses throughout the day, especially after meals. To boost deeper sleep, take right before bedtime. Calcium will have even more impact when taken with some hot milk or hot milk and honey. (Honey helps the body retain fluid and somewhat arrests the need to get up to urinate.)

FOOD SOURCES: Eat all dairy products, bone meal and some green vegeta-bles. (Incidentally, check to make sure your market doesn't sell milk forti-fied with bovine growth hormone. It's not good for you or your children.) For a real sleep-inducer, add a half cup of powdered milk to a quart of milk.

IRON/COPPER

A deficiency of iron or copper may cause insomnia. (The first sign of a copper deficiency is osteoporosis.) However, do not take iron or copper supplements unless prescribed by a nutritionist or knowledgeable physi-cian. It's important to note that vigorous exercise which causes a great deal of perspiration can deplete the body of iron.

FOOD SOURCES: Iron is found in green, leafy vegetables, liver, eggs, fish, meat, poultry, whole grains, avocados, almonds, pumpkins, dried prunes, dates, beets, rice and wheat bran, soybeans, millet, parsley and blackstrap molasses. Copper is widely distributed in such foods as almonds, avocados, barley, beans, beets, nuts, raisins, salmon, soybeans and green, leafy vegetables.

MAGNESIUM

Magnesium is a natural sedative and helps prevent twitching of limbs. Patients who are magnesium-deficient often have insomnia and, as with a calcium deficiency, may find it hard to return to sleep once awakened. With corrective doses of 250 to 300 mg a day, patients report lowered anxiety levels and more uninterrupted, refreshing sleep. Magnesium levels should always be calculated as one part magnesium to two parts of calcium (2:1 ratio). Take divided doses after meals and before bedtime.

FOOD SOURCES: Most foods contain some magnesium. It is found in meat, fish, dairy products and seafood. Other easy sources are apples, apricots, avocados, bananas, brewer's yeast, brown rice, figs, garlic, kelp, lima beans, millet, nuts, peaches, salmon, sesame seeds, tofu, green, leafy vegetables, wheat and whole grains.

TRYPTOPHAN

Eating food or taking supplements with the essential amino acid trypto-phan has a profound effect on sleepiness. One of tryptophan's metabolic duties is to help manufacture the neurotransmitter serotonin, a substance which coaxes us into sleep. Research shows it takes about an hour for tryptophan to reach the brain and be transformed into serotonin. While tryptophan is available in both protein and carbohydrate food sources, carbohydrate intake is more influential in promoting sleepiness.

For years sleep researchers quite successfully used tryptophan supple-ments to induce sleep. However, a few years ago one batch of this amino acid was unfortunately contaminated, and it is presently banned by the FDA, though the ban was partially lifted in 1996 so that physicians can now prescribe tryptophan for those patients who need it.

If you are taking tryptophan, it is important to take it with fruit juice to carry it quickly to the brain. Start out with a dose of 500 mg and increase in 500-mg increments to the cutoff of 2,000 mg, or 2 grams. Take dose one hour before bedtime for three days and then do not take for the next four days. Continue the rhythm of three days on and four days off. To intensify the effect, also take 250 mg niacin, plus high-carbohydrate foods such as wheat bread with peanut butter or a slice of avocado. The supplement is successfully used for PMS and other sleep-related respiratory disturbances.

FOOD SOURCES: A glass of warm milk contains tryptophan, as does a banana and a teaspoon of peanut butter or nut butter. Or you may find it pleasant and helpful to eat half a grapefruit just before going to bed. Other foods high in tryptophan include dates, figs, rice, tuna, turkey and yogurt. The following list shows the amount of tryptophan in sleep-inducing foods:

FOOD	QUANTITY	MG
Tuna	3/4 cup	914
Cottage cheese	1 cup	336
Rice (white)	1 cup	157
Oatmeal (dry)	1 cup	146
Nonfat fortified milk	1 glass	137
Egg	1 large	112
Peanut butter	1 oz	109

VITAMIN B COMPLEX

In general, the entire family of B-complex vitamins controls healthy nerves, is influential in achieving restful sleep and helps prevent insomnia, depression and anxiety. All the B vitamins must first be taken as a family, and then if they are needed, specific B "team" vitamins can also be taken. Stress quickly reduces reserves of B vitamins in the body, and this can cause insomnia. B vitamins are also depleted by smoking, drinking alcohol and taking birth control pills.

Another reason the B-vitamin family is important for sleep is that these vitamins manage the body's use of all amino acids, including sleep-inducing tryptophan. Among the B vitamins that strongly influence sleep are B3 (niacin), B5 (pantothenic acid), B6 (pyridoxine), B12 (cyanocobalamin), folic acid and inositol. Occasionally, some few people have a paradoxical reaction to a B-vitamin regimen, and instead of being helped to go to sleep, they may become more energized.

FOOD SOURCES: Whole grains, which are useful to increase one's sense of tranquility and reduce tension and irritability, are high in B vitamins. Brewer's yeast is high in B-complex vitamins, as are peanuts, walnuts, sunflower seeds and bananas.

B3 (NIACIN)

Niacin helps sleep by extending the impact of the amino acid tryptophan, especially in people with mild depression. It also helps those who fall asleep easily but awaken frequently during the night. However, niacin may cause flushing. The therapeutic dose is 50 to 100 mg a day. Some nutritionists advise 50 mg three times a day.

B5 (PANTOTHENIC ACID)

B5 is useful in preventing stress and may be useful in alleviating symptoms of depression and anxiety. It is required by every cell in the body and helps convert nutrients into energy.

B6 (PYRIDOXINE)

B6, which is a natural sedative and has enormous management responsibilities in the body, regulates tryptophan, magnesium and protein metabolism. The use of oral contraceptives, antidepressants and estrogen increase the need for B6. The therapeutic dose is between 10 to 50 mg a day.

Carpal tunnel syndrome or repetitive strain injury occurs with repetitive finger and wrist work at machinery or computers. It causes pins and needles in the hands and interferes with one's ability to sleep. Three supplements can help overcome carpal tunnel: B6 (50 mg), calcium/magnesium combination (1,000 to 500 mg) and capsules of unsaturated essential fatty acids: borage, black current seed or flaxseed oil. Another element that helps is to have a physiotherapist apply a TENS (transcutaneous electrical neural stimulator) machine. The electrical impulse applications seem to work best on the palm—on the fleshy part of the thumb and the area about one inch down from the ring finger and the pinky.

Food Sources: Bananas, sunflower seeds, peanuts, whole grains and wheat germ are excellent sources of B6.

B12 (CYANOCOBALAMIN)

B12 is essential to the health of the nervous system. It may help restore normal sleep/wake patterns and act as an antistress agent. The normal therapeutic dose is 25 mg daily.

FOOD SOURCES: Milk, eggs, cheese, liver, yeast and wheat germ are all high in B12. Because B12 is not found in vegetables, some strict vegetarians have a B12 deficiency.

FOLIC ACID

A deficiency of folic acid may result in insomnia. Taking supplements of folic acid also helps in the treatment of depression and anxiety. A sore, red tongue is one sign of a folic acid deficiency. Such problems are treated with 2 to 5 mg daily.

INOSITOL

Inositol has been helpful in the treatment of some insomniacs and is often used with 100 mg of B5. While it should not be taken on a regular basis, a 500 to 1000 mg dose of inositol can have a powerful tranquilizing effect. It's best to take a dose one hour before bedtime.

FOOD SOURCES: Brown rice, brewer's yeast, wheat germ, citrus fruit and beef heart are good sources of inositol.

VITAMIN C

Vitamin C encourages restful sleep, helps calm nerves and serves as a prime antioxidant. While the RDA is much lower, therapeutic doses of vitamin C range between 500 and 2000 mg. It is best to divide doses during the day or take a time-release vitamin C.

FOOD SOURCES: Citrus fruits and many vegetables contain vitamin C.

VITAMIN D

Vitamin D regulates calcium and health of the nerves. It should never be taken without calcium. Supplements need to be converted by the liver and kidneys.

FOOD SOURCES: The best sources of vitamin D are fish, such as halibut, cod and tuna, and fish liver oils, especially cod liver oil. Vitamin D is also contained in oatmeal, sardines, egg yolk, butter, alfalfa, sweet potatoes and some vegetable oils. To create vitamin D within the body, expose the face and arms to sunlight about three days a week.

VITAMIN E

Vitamin E, a major antioxidant, has a great many functions within the body. In relation to sleep needs, it helps circulation. The normal dose is 400 IUs per day, but menopausal women and older people may need to take up to 800 IUs daily. Start at 30 IU and work upwards slowly.

FOOD SOURCES: Eat green, leafy vegetables, whole grains, vegetable oils and wheat germ

ZINC

Zinc deficiency can result in insomnia in adults. The RDA for zinc is 15 mg for adults and slightly more for pregnant and nursing women. Zinc can be used separately for several weeks or included in a balanced mineral supplement. If an infant is deficient in zinc, it may show up in frequent awakenings and crying.

FOOD SOURCES: Brewer's yeast, wheat germ, nuts, seeds, fish oil, whole grains, pumpkin seeds, pecans, sardines, sunflower seeds, as well as meats, poultry, seafood and oysters are excellent sources of this vital nutrient.

Natural Sleep Remedies for Adults

Sleeplessness becomes insomnia when a person develops a pattern of sleeping without being rested and a recurring mode of not being able to sleep despite fatigue and sleepiness.

Natural remedies have all proven to be very successful in curing adult insomnia. They include (1) elimination of certain stimulating foods, (2) eating sleep-provoking foods, (3) the use of key relaxing and hypnotic mind exercises, (4) the judicious use of safe, sedative herbal teas and Bach flower remedies, (5) application of water to promote total relaxation and (6) the use of specific safe, natural homeopathic and biochemical tissue salts. (For a discussion of water therapies, see Chapter 9; for a discussion of physical and mental exercises, see Chapter 10.) The following chart lists various sleep problems and the many different kinds of natural remedies you can use to solve them. But first a brief description of homeopathic remedies and tissue salts is needed. For a thorough discussion of both these topics, see Chapter 8.

In the homeopathic system of medicine, like cures like. Just as insect stings are cured with homeopathic pills derived from honeybees, a key cause of insomnia, coffee, is the effective homeopathic cure for sleeplessness, restlessness and excessive mental activity. Derived from the coffee bean, Coffea is produced from unroasted coffee beans that are diluted greatly according to strict homeopathic standards. Dosage is one pill dissolved under the tongue. Discontinue the remedy as soon as the problem is alleviated. If the first remedy in the following chart doesn't work, try another one that matches the symptoms. Homeopathic effectiveness depends on closely matching symptoms with the remedy, taking the lowest dosage possible and activating one's own inner healing abilities.

Tissue salts are another natural remedy. According to homeopaths who

have used such biochemical substances since the late 1800s, "sleep disturbances are caused primarily by alterations in the balance of mineral salts
in the tissues of the brain and nervous system." Of the twelve tissue salts,
the following are the most important for insomnia: Ferrum Phos., Kali
Phos., Natrum Mur., Natrum Sulph. and Magnesia Phos.

At-a-Glance Chart of Adult Natural Sleep Remedies

To cure chronic (long-standing) insomnia, take one homeopathic tablet
marked either 6c or 6x under the tongue (do not chew it) three times a day
for up to fourteen days. To cure acute or emergency insomnia, generally take
one homeopathic tablet marked 30c or 30x every twelve hours for several
days. (Because of pollution homeopaths in many European countries now
advise taking higher dosages—3 to 5 tablets—than usually recommended in
Great Britain or the United States.) Unless otherwise noted, adults should take
five tissue salts under the tongue or dissolved in water every two hours. Take
less frequently as the condition improves. When two different tissue salts are
mentioned, use them alternately on an hourly basis. For severe cases, dissolve
the salts in hot water. Discontinue the tissue salt remedy once the problem
is alleviated.

**Note that throughout the chart the abbreviation H stands for homeo-
pathic remedy and TS stands for tissue salts. Dosage sizes have been
abbreviated to read, for example, "6c/x"; however, when buying them,
you should ask for either 6c or 6x.**

PROBLEM	COPING STRATEGIES
CHRONIC INSOMNIA Difficult time falling asleep or, once awakened, falling back to sleep.	• Practice sleep mindfulness (see Chapter 10). • Eliminate coffee and caffeinated tea. Drink sedative herbal tea daily (see Chapter 8). • Take a leisurely full hot bath (see Chapter 9). Passive heat first raises, then lowers body temperature and produces quiet drowsiness. • Immerse feet in shallow hot foot bath. This diverts blood from head to produce drowsiness.

PROBLEM	COPING STRATEGIES
	• Apply hot moist compresses to head or lower spine. • Occasionally apply a cold abdominal compress (called "Neptune's Girdle"). This diverts blood from head to trunk and produces drowsiness.
CHRONIC AND/OR OCCASIONAL INSOMNIA	Long-range water revitalization therapies, including daily cold water treatments, harden the body, increase resistance to disease and create a feeling of well-being. • Cold water treading: Place toes under cold running water, gradually increasing tolerance to the cold water. Eventually tread (walk) in cold water up to several minutes. • Friction rubs: Occasionally rub the entire body with a cold, wet crocheted mitten or loofah. Occasionally use coarse salt as a friction rub on the upper parts of the body during bath or shower.
TIRED Need a good night's sleep.	• Take a 15-minute neutral temperature bath. • Or take a sedative full hot bath.
Fall asleep too early: phase-advanced sleep syndrome.	• Hot baths. • Herbal sleep inducers. • Variety of tissue salts. • Take 0.5 mg of melatonin upon awakening in the middle of the night. • Deliberately change sleep routine.
SLEEPLESSNESS Inability to fall asleep. Mild case.	• Apply hot moist compress to head for a few minutes. Direct application of heat to head creates drowsiness.

PROBLEM	COPING STRATEGIES
	• Hot foot bath: Run several inches of hot water in bathtub and place feet in water for a few minutes. This diverts blood from head and creates drowsiness.
Fall asleep too late (anytime after midnight): this is a phase-delayed sleep syndrome.	• Take any of the homeopathic and/or tissue salts suggested for sleeplessness. • In addition, take the following doses of melatonin: For one week, take 0.5 to 1 mg 2 hours before current bedtime. For next 3 days to 1 week, take dosage 2½ hours before old bedtime. Move time back by a half hour every 3 days (to a week) until you have reached desired bedtime.
Can never sleep before midnight.	• 5 tablets TS 6c/x Calcarea Sulph. 3 times daily for 2 weeks or 1 tablet H 30c/x Coffea 1 hour before desired bedtime for 10 nights. • 1 tablet H 30c/x Pulsatilla 1 hour before bedtime for 10 nights.
Sleepless after midnight.	• 5 tablets TS 6c/x Silica. • 1 tablet H 30c/x Coffea or Nux Vomica 1 hour before bedtime every night for 10 nights.
Sleepless between 1 and 2 A.M.	• 1 tablet H 6c/x Kali Carb. or, if chronic condition, a 30c/x dose 1 hour before desired bedtime for 10 days. Repeat if awakened.
Sleepless after 3 or 4 A.M.	• 1 tablet H 6c/x Sulphur or, if chronic condition, 1 tablet 30c/x before bedtime for 10 days. Repeat dose if awakened.

PROBLEM	COPING STRATEGIES
Sleepless from nervous causes.	• 5 tablets TS 6c/x Kali Phos.
Sleepless from excitement.	• 5 tablets TS 6c/x Ferrum Phos. and Nat. Phos. • 1 tablet H 30c/x Lycopedium when the mind is overactive before going to bed, there is considerable worrying about events of day and you can't fall asleep until morning.
Sleepless and unable to calm down; can be from joy, overexcitement or bad news.	• 1 tablet H 30c/x Coffea before bedtime for 10 nights. If you awaken and can't get back to sleep, repeat dose.
Sleepless with fear and great nervousness.	• 1 tablet H 30c/x Aconite one hour before bedtime for 10 nights. Repeat dose if awakened and cannot fall back asleep
Constant worry interferes with sleep (might be future events in office, school, for family or friends or possibility of nightmare).	• 5 tablets TS 6c/x Ferrum Phos.
Sleeplessness due to too much studying or thinking.	• Water therapies (also effective for treating head colds): (1) To relieve head congestion: Take brief hot foot bath. Occasionally follow with tonic alternate hot and cold stream to the bottom of the feet. (2) Put on sedative cold wet stockings, cover with dry wool stockings. This diverts congestion to feet so brain relaxes and starts to feel drowsy. • 1 tablet H 30c/x Nux Vomica good for intense overwork, overstudying and especially if one cannot sleep before midnight and awakens between 2 and 3 A.M.

PROBLEM	COPING STRATEGIES
PROBLEMS DURING SLEEP Restless sleep.	• 1 tablet H 30c/x Passiflora. If general problem, especially if caused by overactive mind filled with worries and ideas, take one hour before bedtime for ten nights.
Sleepwalking.	• 5 tablets TS 6c/x Kali Phos. 3 times daily as needed.
Grits teeth during sleep.	• 5 tablets TS 6c/x Nat. Phos. 3 times daily.
Starts (involuntary moves) during sleep.	• 5 tablets TS 6c/x Nat. Mur. 3 times daily.
Muscles twitch before falling asleep.	• 5 tablets TS 6c/x Kali Phos.
Muscles twitch during sleep.	• 5 tablets TS 6c/x Nat. Sulph.
Irritability results in insomnia. (Also useful if overresponsive to noise and feels critical of everyone else.)	• If chronic, 1 tablet H 6c/x Nux Vomica several times a day. If acute, use 30c/x 1 hour before bedtime. Repeat dose if awakened.
Awakened by flatulence (gas).	• 5 tablets TS 6c/x Nat. Sulph. every 2 hours. If chronic, take 3 times a day until relief is achieved. • If chronic, drink small amounts of tea made from these anti-gas herbs until relief: bruised, strained caraway, anise or dill seeds. Other helpful herb teas: chamomile flowers, peppermint leaves, Melissa (lemon balm). • Take activated charcoal tablets (sold in drugstores) to absorb gas and/or food poisons.

PROBLEM	COPING STRATEGIES
Awakened during the night and cannot go back to sleep.	• If frequent, immerse the lower part of the body in a shallow (6-to 8-inch) cold shallow (sitz) bath 2 to 3 times a week.
Light sleepers who react to every disturbance.	• 1 tablet H 6c/x Ignatia 3 times daily for 10 days. • For hypersensitivity to sound, 1 tablet H 6c/x Coffea 3 times daily.
Pain from nonemerging wisdom tooth or teeth (other symptoms may be swollen gums, swollen glands in the neck, sore throat that makes it hard to swallow).	• 5 tablets TS 6c/x Silica helps teeth cut through so lancing is not necessary.
DREAMS Sleep problems during dreams. Anxious, deep, heavy dreams.	• 5 tablets TS 6c/x Nat. Sulph.
Exclamations during sleep and dreams or frequent dreams.	• 5 tablets TS 6c/x Silica.
Dreams perceived as too vivid.	• 5 tablets TS 6c/x Calcarea Phos.
Shock from an injury creates tendency for bad dreams.	• 1 tablet H 6c/x Arnica 4 times daily up to 14 days. N.B.: Arnica, made from a yellow mountain flower, is remedy of choice for any injury. In addition to taking pills that are easily dissolved under the tongue, Arnica ointment can safely be applied to area of injury, if skin is unbroken.
NIGHTMARES Nightmares with tossing, turning and great fear.	• 1 tablet H 30c/x Aconite 1 hour before bedtime for 10 nights. If awakened, repeat dose.

PROBLEM	COPING STRATEGIES
Nightmares that cause incontinence.	• 1 tablet H 6c/x Equisetum for 14 nights.
Nightmares with indigestion.	• Alternate 5 tablets TS 6c/x Kali Sulph. and Nat. Sulph. as long as condition continues.
SLEEPINESS Constant need to sleep longer in morning.	• 5 tablets TS 6c/x Nat. Mur. Repeat 3 times daily until problem lessens or disappears.
Sleepy in the morning.	• 5 tablets TS 6c/x Nat. Sulph. if situation just crops up. If chronic, repeat dose 3 times daily for extended period.
Hard time waking up or being awakened in the morning.	• 5 tablets TS 6c/x Calcarea Phos. for either chronic or acute condition.
Sleepy in the afternoon.	• 1 tablet H 6c/x Sulphur. If chronic, take 3 times daily for 10 to 14 days.
Sleepy after meals.	• 1 tablet H 6c/x Nux Vomica. If chronic, repeat dose 3 times daily for 10 to 14 days.
Unusually sleepy in warm weather.	• 5 tablets TS 6c/x Nat. Mur. If chronic, repeat dose 3 times daily for 10 to 14 days. (Deficiency of Nat. Mur. causes disturbances of water in the body. Taking Nat. Mur. distributes water throughout the body.)
DROWSINESS Sleepy and drowsy in the afternoon.	• 5 tablets TS 6c/x Ferrum Phos.
Drowsy because of fever, but still can't get to sleep at night.	• 5 tablets TS 6c/x Ferrum Phos.

Problem	Coping Strategies
Drowsy during the day because of stomach problems or indigestion.	• 5 tablets TS 6c/x Nat. Sulph. every 3 to 4 hours. (Take Nat. Sulph. for digestive problems. It assists in last stages of digestion and also helps dispose of body wastes.)
Restless, unrefreshed sleep: Tired in the morning, strong desire to sleep.	• 5 tablets 6x Nat. Mur. Repeat dose 3 times daily for several weeks.
INAPPROPRIATE WAKEFULNESS Generally feel awake when it is time to go to sleep.	• Alternate 5 tablets TS 6c/x Kali Phos. and Ferrum Phos. 3 times daily for about 2 weeks.
Usually awaken about 3 or 4 A.M. and can't fall asleep until dawn. Wake up tired.	• 1 tablet H 30c/x Nux Vomica one hour before bedtime for 10 nights. Repeat dose if awakened again and can't fall back to sleep.
Can't fall asleep or get back to sleep because can't stop thinking.	• 1 tablet H 6c/x Coffea. • Try Bach flower remedy White Chestnut, which is specifically for thoughts that continue as if on a merry-go-round. Take a few drops under the tongue, or add 3 to 4 drops to water and drink.
Can only sleep in short spurts during the night; get up feeling unrejuvenated.	• 1 tablet H 6c/x Phosphorus every 3 to 4 hours for 2 weeks.
JET LAG	Melatonin therapy: See section on jet lag (Chapter 2) for method of administering melatonin. Warnings on who should not take it and how to choose it are at the end of this chart.

Problem	Coping Strategies
General.	Drink one glass of water for every hour in the air. Walk and stretch as often as possible. Do not drink alcohol or coffee. Adopt local time as soon as you arrive.
Flying east.	Leave early in the day.
Flying west.	Fly late in the day.
WINTER BLUES OR DEPRESSION Phase-delayed sleep syndrome.	Exceptionally bright light between 6 and 9 A.M. fools the body into thinking it isn't a short winter day but a long spring day. Seek treatment at a sleep disorders center, or use high intensity lamps (see Resources). If neither is available, take a walk between 6 and 9 A.M.

What about Taking Melatonin Supplements?

According to sleep researchers the impact of melatonin supplementation varies from person to person. Some people react to melatonin within a half hour. Others take up to two and a half hours to feel its influence.

At the annual American Psychiatric Association meeting in New York in 1996, Dr. Lewy of the Sleep Disorders Research Section at Oregon Health Sciences University in Portland explained to physicians that they could prescribe melatonin to be taken one or two hours before the patient's normal or desired bedtime. He further explained how research scientists determine the beginning of a person's melatonin secretion. For most people melatonin onset is fourteen hours after their circadian time zero, which is usually (but not always) at 7 A.M. This means that most people start producing melatonin about 9 P.M. at night. That is why sleep experts usually suggest patients take melatonin two hours before the anticipated sleep "delivery" time (exceptions are when the body clock must be "reshifted" and "managed"). (People with serious insomnia can go to a sleep clinic or to sleep specialists to have their blood and their saliva assayed to find the exact amount and timing of their melatonin secretion.)

Because the amount of melatonin the body manufactures and needs is so small—a picogram—which is a millionth of a millionth of a gram, Dr. Lewy and other researchers suggest physicians start their patients at the lowest possible dose, working upwards from 0.5 to 3 mg (sometimes, but more rarely, up to 5 mg). In fact, Lewy and others only use half a milligram (0.5) for jet lag, winter depression and advanced and delay phase sleep problems. The team headed by Dr. Richard Wurtman at MIT showed excellent results for sleep management, jet lag and clock irregularities with an even smaller amount of 0.3 mg. Dr. Lewy notes that each dose is excreted within several hours from the body. When melatonin is taken for sleep or shift-phasing purposes, Dr. Lewy adds that it is useful for the patient to wear a sleep mask and/or to keep the sleeping room dark.

WARNINGS ABOUT MELATONIN USE

Though melatonin is widely touted as the great cureall for sleeplessness, researchers advise that it should be used cautiously, taking the following conditions into consideration:

- Additives: Always read the label carefully to avoid unwanted wheat, gluten, egg, milk or animal derivatives. Also check for such inactive ingredients as corn or rice starch, gelatin, methycellulose or talc.
- Children: There have been various successful studies of overstimulated children who have been given small amounts of melatonin to help them sleep. Nevertheless, Dr. Lewy advises caution and only short-term administration of melatonin, since toxicity and other side effects have not been determined.
- Depression: Unless you are under the direct supervision of a physician, melatonin is contraindicated for people who have had episodes of depression or have a family history which includes depression.
- Diseases: People with diabetes, depression, epilepsy, eye diseases such as retinitis pigmentosa, leukemia and migraine headaches should avoid melatonin. Also keep away from melatonin if you have an autoimmune disease such as rheumatoid arthritis. The jury is still out on whether or not melatonin can increase immunity. Obviously, if it does, you don't want to aggravate any autoimmune problem.
- Jet lag: See Chapter 2.
- Job alertness: Unless you are under a physician's supervision do not use melatonin if handling heavy machinery, driving a truck, flying a plane or working as an engineer on the railroad or subway.
- Medicines: Medicines of various kinds increase or decrease the melatonin secreted by the body. For example, caffeine and nonsteroidal anti-

inflammatory drugs are known to lower the amount of melatonin manufactured by the body. If you are on prescription medicines or oral contraceptives, consult your physician before taking melatonin on your own so that she can check to see how melatonin influences these drugs.

- Nightmares: Anecdotal information indicates that melatonin may increase the vividness of dreams.
- Sleep apnea: Sleep researchers don't think melatonin will be useful for sleep apnea or restless legs.
- Winter depression: See Chapter 2.

If you cannot take melatonin, experts at your local sleep disorders clinic can easily address any problems and help you reset an errant clock.

Who Should Not Take Melatonin

Research shows melatonin should not be taken by the following people:

- Women who are considering getting pregnant.
- Pregnant women.
- Breast-feeding women.
- People with autoimmune diseases, diabetes, epilepsy, leukemia or migraine headaches.
- Anyone with a tendency for depression.
- Anyone who is already taking an antidepressant.

POSSIBLE SIDE EFFECTS

Of course, side effects vary from person to person, and there is always the possibility of personal sensitivity to a product. There have been some reports that a small group of people get sleepy immediately after taking the hormone. To avoid this possible reaction, do not drive yourself to the airport if you take melatonin at home before a long-distance plane ride. About eight out of 100 people have a paradoxical reaction to melatonin: Instead of getting sleepy at nighttime, they get sleepy during the day. And two out of 100 people experience minor nausea, headache, giddiness or fuzzy thinking.

TYPES OF MELATONIN TO PURCHASE

Investigators working with melatonin have discovered that there is a disadvantage in melatonin not being regulated by the Food and Drug Administration (FDA). They have found considerable differences between various products, some containing little or no melatonin, some containing additives and impurities and at least one containing a sleeping pill. Since there are no standards for purity, products vary from company to company. When CNN did an overview of the melatonin phenomenon, their investigators discovered many over-the-counter pills were not accurate in the amount of milligrams listed.

Remember it's best to buy only synthetically manufactured supplements. Do not buy the following:

- Sustained-release melatonin, which may have a contradictory effect than that desired.
- Bovine pineal gland extracts. Do not be influenced by the fact that they may be sold as "natural" products. Researchers such as Dr. Lewy recommend that due to the current fear of transmittable viruses and possible contamination from mad cow disease, all unheated and untreated cow substances should be avoided. Such cow substances have been banned in Canada, Europe and Great Britain.

Fortunately, most melatonin marketed in the United States is made from synthetic sources. However, university sleep researchers bemoan the fact that there are no strict standards for the manufacture of melatonin, except for laboratory use. One MIT researcher believes only laboratory melatonin is pure enough to use. It's important to note that sleep clinics have access to reliable sources of melatonin.

PART

II

Children's Sleep Problems
and Solutions

Sleep is a natural function. It is important for parents to know that falling asleep is not just one event but rather a series of consecutive events which vary between initial drowsiness to light sleep into deep sleep, with brief arousals between deep sleep and dream sleep. During this time it is normal for the child to awaken briefly and even stare with a blank look, to toss and turn and at some period to even briefly awaken to check the covers, toys and room. It is essential for each child to find his or her own way and comfort in falling asleep again after waking up. Child sleeping problems usually occur if the child gets used to always being helped—rocked, walked, sung to or fed—when he or she wakes up. A child who is always helped, and cannot manage to fall asleep without help, will not discover that it is possible to fall asleep on his or her own.

Laboratory investigations show that children already evidence stages of sleep in utero, although infants are born with only a primitive version of NREM (nondreaming) sleep. After about the third month NREM sleep gradually develops its characteristic four stages (see Chapter 1 for a thorough discussion of the four stages). Each stage of childhood—infant, toddler, school child, teen—has its own sleep needs (see the Children's

Average Sleep Chart). How to deal,with special problems of sleeplessness (unwillingness or inability to go to sleep) or wakefulness when aroused from sleep is addressed for each age group in Chapters 5 through 7 in this part of the book.

However, it must be stressed that children are born with different sleep needs. Laboratory tests show the normal range of sleep, but these are approximate. Lifelong traits of being an early person (a lark) or an evening

Approximate Average Sleep Needs: Infancy to Late Adolescence

HRS	WK 1	MO 1	MO 3	MO 6	MO 9	YR 1	YR 1½	YR 2	YR 3	YR 4	YR 5
1											
2											
3											
4											
5											
6											
7											
8											
9											
10											
11											
12											
13											
14											
15											
16											
17											
TOTAL SLEEP HRS	16½	15½	15	14¼	14	13¾	13½	13	12	11½	11

NIGHT TIME SLEEP ■   DAYTIME SLEEP 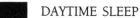 ■

person (an owl) reveal themselves early in a child's life. Whatever the child's disposition, it helps to realize that children who get enough sleep tend to be less moody, recuperate faster after an illness and develop stronger memory and concentration skills. If your child varies considerably from the known norms, you might consider discussing his specific needs with a sleep or pediatric professional.

YR 6	YR 7	YR 8	YR 9	YR 10	YR 11	YR 12	YR 13	YR 14	YR 15	YR 16	YR 17	YR 18
10 3/4	10 1/2	10 1/4	10	9 3/4	9 1/2	9 1/4	9 1/4	9	8 3/4	8 1/2	8 1/4	8 1/4

Parents' Sleep Pact

Sleep is a time of isolation and separation from the family. It is essential that it never be used as a punishment for a child and that an integrated family routine be developed between the child and the parents or caregivers. The following Parents' Sleep Pact, which I devised especially for this book, is filled with simple concepts and time-honored routines that can help parents avert present and future sleep problems for their children.

- Create a dependable, yet flexible mealtime, naptime and sleeptime that coincides with family needs.
- In order to relieve your child of present or future nighttime anxiety and sleep problems, pledge to avoid black moods, impatience, indignation, irritability and toss away fatigue, boredom, anger and other personal cares when you feed your child and prepare to put her to bed.
- Each night, and all nights of your child's early life, establish a happy, consistent and memorable routine at bedtime.
- If possible, provide a ten-minute transition period for yourself between your daytime routine and putting your child to bed. During the transition try to sit quietly and breathe deeply, meditate or take an invigorating, restorative shower.
- Each night create a bedtime oasis of calm. Establish a quiet period of smiles, cooing and happy interaction. Do not instigate horseplay, tickling or stimulating activities. Put your child to bed with pleasure, firmness and kindliness.
- Whenever possible, devote at least ten minutes to giving your child a warm, relaxing and fun bath. Remember that warm baths tranquilize crying and irritable children.
- From infancy onward read a soothing, comforting, lulling bedtime story to your child.
- Each morning be mindful about your first greeting to your child, so that he will anticipate a pleasant, happy day ahead.

5

Infant to Toddler Behavior,
Parental Responses

I'll never forget a tired parent of a newborn telling me, "People who say they sleep like a baby obviously don't have one!" While some kids are perfect sleepers from the start, others have to be coaxed into good sleep habits. Because sleep is a series of recurring and repeated stages of light sleep and deeper sleep, it is normal for a newborn to sleep about sixteen or seventeen hours in five installments, but to awaken often and to yawn, fidget, twist, make quiet sounds or fast sucking motions, have eyes dart around under eyelids and maybe even smile. Over three quarters of a newborn's sleep is shallow and light, and the infant is easily awakened during these stages. Usually by three to four months most children are able to sleep most of the night in a successive pattern of five to nine hours. By the end of the first year, most children will be sleeping about 12 to 14 hours. This includes one long period at night and one morning and one afternoon nap.

An important factor in children's ability to sleep is for parents to become aware of their inborn temperament and to understand the process and goals of sleep. Problems may develop during infancy because of children's innate temperament—their predisposition to specific reactions to life, people and events. These personality reactions can have a profound effect on children's ability to sleep and, indeed, on the course of their whole lives. (See the important discussion of the sleep/temperament connection in children in the Appendix.)

Stages of Sleep in Infants to Toddlers

Age	What's Happening	Time Frame	Special/ Dream Facts	Eyes	Brain Activity	Muscles	Heart & Breathing	Temperature	Misc. Facts
FETUS	REM/active sleep	Earliest stage forms at 6–7 months. Firmly established by end of 8th month.	Sleep patterns begin even before birth.	Practices eye movements. May be laying down sensory pathways to sights, sounds and perhaps dream imagery.	• May be important development of brain cells during this activity. • May be important for development of higher brain centers.		Respiration practiced.		
	NREM/ quiet sleep	Occurs 7-8 months. Firmly established at end of 8th month.			Requires certain degree of brain maturation.		No breathing motions.		

NEWBORN	REM/active sleep	• Sleeps about 16-17 hours a day, a few hours at a time. About 5 to 7 sleeping and waking periods throughout day/night. • Up to one month enters REM immediately after falling asleep.	Dreams only occur in REM sleep.	Eyes dart back and forth under eyelids.	More blood flows to brain.	Twitches.; may smile briefly; poor muscle tone.	Both irregular.	Regulation impaired, though no sweating or shivering. Body uses more oxygen because it is spending more energy.	Premature babies spend 80% sleeeptime in REM. Full-term infants spend 50% sleeptime in REM. Need for REM sleep gets progressively less, continuing to late adolescence and adulthood when only 25% sleeptime in REM.

Stages of Sleep in Infants to Toddlers (continued)

Age	What's Happening	Time Frame	Special/Dream Facts	Eyes	Brain Activity	Muscles	Heart & Breathing	Temperature	Misc. Facts
NEWBORN (continued)	NREM/quiet sleep	NREM sleep develops into four stages: (1) drowsiness, (2) light sleep, (3) transition to deeper sleep, (4) delta sleep.				Lies very still; occasionally body jerks or sudden motion startles. This reaction disappears during first month.	Breathes deeply.		Full-term infants spend 50% sleeptime in NREM.

| THREE MONTHS | REM sleep | Sleep approx. 15 hours a day in 4-5 sleep periods. Between 3-6 months baby should be sleeping most of the night from last feeding to early morning awakening. | Spend only 33% of sleeptime in REM. First REM brief, then into NREM with quick descent into (4) deep sleep. After 40-50 minutes another arousal, followed by 5 to 20-minute REM. Then another arousal. | Checks to see if everything is okay. | Moves about, goes back to sleep. | Awakenings throughout night very normal. Important for muscles, joints, skin, and reassurance that things are normal. |

Stages of Sleep in Infants to Toddlers (continued)

Age	What's Happening	Time Frame	Special/Dream Facts	Eyes	Brain Activity	Muscles	Heart & Breathing	Temperature	Misc. Facts
THREE MONTHS (continued)	NREM sleep • Abnormal behavior: confusion, thrashing.	10-minute plunge through (1) drowsy to (4) deep sleep, which lasts one hour; brief few seconds to several minute arousal; then return to sleep.	Now enters NREM sleep first. This pattern continues throughout life.	During arousal eyes may open with blank stare.		During arousal may move suddenly, cry, turn over.			Child in stage 4 sleep impossible to awaken.

SIX MONTHS	Sleep schedule and consecutive nighttime sleep should be resolved.	Sleep about 12 hours a night with brief awakenings. Take 1-2 hour naps in mid-morning and afternoon.
ONE YEAR		• Sleep about 14 hours. • May give up morning nap by 2.
TWO YEARS		• Sleep 11-12 hours. • 1-2 hour nap after lunch.

Common Infant to Toddler Sleep Problems

The lucky child is born with a mature nervous system and a fully developed digestive system so he goes about the first months of life happily eating and sleeping. However, numerous newborns have trouble falling asleep or getting back to sleep. Parents everywhere in the world, through kindliness and often with a sense of exhausted desperation, allow their child to steer them through the first maze of eating and sleeping. Often enough, the kind gesture gets to be the very thing the child demands to have repeated. Fortunately, the ability to fall asleep, if not inborn, can be learned through routine or guided responses.

No one actually knows all the reasons a newborn will sleep poorly, although two strong possibilities are undeveloped nervous or digestive systems. These can lead to agitated and crampy crying, often called "colic," in the first weeks of life. Another cause may be an allergy to milk and other lactose products. If you suspect such a sensitivity, immediately eliminate cow's milk from the diet of the nursing mother or replace cow's milk with a soy formula or goat's milk for bottle-fed children. Mothers who are having trouble nursing should contact a local chapter or the national office of the La Leche League and also reach out for advice and help to other nearby nursing mothers.

It may help to remember that lusty crying, while hard on a parent's nerves, is a good sign that the child has a set of healthy lungs. However, as experience will prove again and again, not all crying is about hunger. Smiling, cooing, stroking, caressing, singing and humming lullabies and other gentle favorite songs, deliberate eye connection and talking and saying nonsense words make the newborn feel safe and loved. While all these activities have been shown to increase neuron connections in the brain and help the child in its life-long struggle with self-identity and trust, they are also strongly connected to how well and when a child sleeps.

A study shows that white noise which duplicates sounds in the uterus can calm babies to sleep. Twenty newborns several days old slept with a white noise device placed 12 to 20 inches from their heads. Sixteen of the twenty fell into a restful sleep within five minutes. These findings show that white noise is useful in calming babies who have difficulties falling asleep. (See Resources for various infant sleep aids.)

A study on the connection between room temperature and waking up at night shows cooler rooms and less bundling of children can help those who awake often during the night. Researchers theorize that a baby must expend a considerable amount of metabolic effort on proper temperature regulation. In a hot room, with warm wraps, the effort may create so much stress that the baby becomes uncomfortable and wakes up.

In the past, most parents, even those who carry their children on their backs, put them to sleep on their stomachs. But physicians have discovered that this allows some vulnerable babies, in fact, some 5,000 to 6,000 American babies a year, to succumb to the fatal breathing disorder called "sudden infant death" (SID). A recent "back-to-sleep movement" initiated by the National Institute of Child Health and Human Development (NICHHD) urged parents not to put children to sleep on their stomachs but on their backs or sides. This awareness has prevented almost half of the usual number of SID deaths. However, if infants aren't comfortable on their backs or sides, parents can provide some supportive pillow aids to ensure children's comfort. (Mail order sources are listed in the Resources.)

Is having children sleep in the parents' bed a good idea or not? Throughout early civilization and in most nonWestern societies, children were encouraged to sleep with parents for warmth and protection. To this day, many anthropologists and parents and some pediatricians revel in the closeness and bonding the "family bed" offers. But in the last several hundred years, and especially during the last seventy-five years, this concept has been put aside, mainly for the child's sake. This is because a host of difficult-to-overcome sleeping problems have emerged when children cannot sleep alone but only in the same bed with parents.

Most pediatric sleep specialists now say the most difficult and prevalent

Tips to Help Establish Good Lifelong Sleep Habits

- Program the day as alert waketime and the night as sleeptime.
- Prepare the infant for bed by establishing a beloved routine and be consistent about the rules.
- Alert your older child about five or ten minutes before bedtime. This gives him time to finish whatever he's doing and helps prepare him for bedtime.
- Put your child to bed awake in a dark, quiet room.
- After finishing a bedtime story, turn the reading lamp to low, turn on a small nightlight or install a gradual dimmer than turns the light off after fifteen minutes.
- Maintain quiet, hushed tones at night.
- Avoid bright lights during nighttime awakenings by placing cool high-tech blue or green nightlights in hallway, bathroom and child's room (see Resources).

childhood sleep problems occur from the inability of some children to get to sleep on their own. That doesn't mean you can't or shouldn't ever cuddle and hold children when they cry out for you during the night. It does mean a young sleep-deprived parent should be on the alert for a prolonged bad sleep pattern which can emerge when their persistently crying newborn will only fall asleep if carried, held, rocked to sleep or allowed to sleep in bed with them. These loving acts can unintentionally lead to negative results. The inability to fall asleep alone may develop into a handicap, and other sleep problems may emerge as an infant moves from one growth stage to the next.

Scenarios to Help Your Infant to Toddler Sleep

How can parents solve some of the many problems that occur when putting infants to sleep? Transforming a difficult situation is hard work, but as a Chinese proverb says: "If we don't change our direction, we are likely to end up where we are headed." Ann Landers put it wonderfully: "Success is the place in the road where preparation and opportunity meet. But too few people recognize it, because too often it comes disguised as hard work."

Included in each of the following scenarios is a parental approach and dialogue as well as proven step-by-step training concepts (also known as behavior modification) to conquer specific sleep problems. The success of the scenarios depends on your patience, persistence and determination to turn any given bad sleep situation around. Though the simple techniques have been found to work for most parents and children, please note that nothing is written in stone. If you find something difficult or unsuited to your child's personality, be creative. Adjust the scenario. Follow your own judgment and instincts when they seem right. Also check the At-a-Glance Chart at the end of the chapter for quick homeopathic remedies, water therapies and other natural cures.

MY NEWBORN DEMANDS TO BE NURSED OR BOTTLE-FED EVERY HOUR THROUGHOUT THE NIGHT

Breastfeeding is a unique and loving experience that can deepen the bond between mother and child. Moreover, it passes the mother's own immunity on to the child. But what can a mother do when she is caught in the revolving door of nursing on demand all through the night? Pretty soon the new mother (or the father if the baby is being bottle-fed) is exhausted and sleep deprived. However, this exhaustion and irritability is but one part of the ongoing problem. Babies who demand on-the-hour feeding, for whatever reason, may be starting a potential sleep problem.

From birth onward every loving smile, soothing touch, eye contact, holding, feeding and bathing experience sets up some valued new hard wiring in the infant's brain. It's much like a computer under construction. Minute by minute, primarily in certain key early months, your child is developing what will eventually be 100 billion neuron and 100 trillion brain connections in the adult brain. When a child is breast-fed or bottle-fed continuously, the circuitry is establishing imperative associations between the act of feeding and sleep, particularly between interrupted sleep and eating. This situation imposes a shaky later sleep routine. It is also possible that a baby being fed that often is consuming too much fluid.

The Solution

After the first few months, you can gradually change the sleep/feeding dialogue between you and your child and teach your baby not to always associate sleep with eating or connect nursing with falling asleep. It is not necessary to wean a baby to separate the association of sleep with nursing. You can easily establish a new, comfortable, normal feeding schedule gradually over the course of the next months.

Pediatric sleep specialists say you can change the time of nursing. Instead of nursing at bedtime, nurse earlier in the day, well before naptime. Keeping the baby's comfort level and sucking ability in mind, gradually increase the time between feedings, progressively adding fifteen minutes at a time. Slowly extend the time between feedings to an hour and a half, and proceed each day until you eventually achieve two hours or two and a half hours between feedings.

When the child begins to fall asleep, disengage the baby by placing your finger at the side of the baby's mouth and withdrawing the nipple. You may, if you want, hold your finger there briefly as the child falls back to sleep. If you are determined to modify your child's waking habits during the night, immediately place the child back in the crib. Changes in the baby's behavior will come about with your consistency and calm reassurance. Even if you have to hide behind the door, make sure your beloved infant falls asleep while you are out of the room.

To assist in behavior modification, you can give your infant a safe homeopathic tissue salt known to cure infants who have a constant need to nurse. Crush one tablet of 6c/x Calc. Phos. tissue salt into a tablespoon of water. Give it to him in an eye dropper. (For a thorough discussion of tissue salts see Chapter 8. Note that you can buy them in either 6c or 6x sizes, which are abbreviated here as 6c/x.)

MY INFANT OVERRESPONDS TO LIGHT IN THE MORNING

By the age of three to four months most children have adjusted their own 24-hour schedule to incorporate light during the day, routine daytime activity in the house as well as the quiet and dark of nighttime. However, many children show a strong sensitivity to daylight and wake up with the first rays of light in their room.

The Solution

Reduce the light in the room with shades that mimic darkness. It may also be necessary to add an additional layer of light-resistant drapes or, if a child is sleeping with other children, to rig up a screen with an awning to shield out light as well as noise.

MY INFANT OVERRESPONDS TO NOISE

Most infants begin to adjust on their own to external cues of quiet, darkness and lack of activity during the night. Many should be on their own 24-hour biological clock by three to four months. However, some noise-sensitive infants react strongly to traffic and various household and people sounds.

The Solution

If you think traffic and other outside noises are influencing the infant's fragmented sleep, you have several choices. Can you move the child to another less noisy section of the house? If not, you can insulate the room with heavy drapes that can be drawn at night. Or try surrounding the child with a screen or improvise a hospital-like curtain around the crib. White-noise machines are a crutch, but they will insulate the child. Two ways to duplicate white noise are putting the radio on between two FM stations or running a vaporizer. Some parents have found the following useful: playing a cassette of lullabies, classical music, the sounds of a summer night in a cornfield or the intriguing, lulling sounds heard on a sailboat in the surf. If the infant is colicky, you might want to investigate machines that duplicate the sound the baby heard in the womb (see Resources).

The homeopathic remedy 3c/x or 6c/x Nux Vomica is useful for worried, anxious, irritable children, especially if they are sensitive to noise and irritated by any disruption or disturbance. Crush one tablet in a tablespoon of water until it dissolves and feed it to the child in an eye dropper about two times a day for ten days to two weeks. This remedy also works for

Making the Transition from Workplace to Child Caregiving

Bach flower remedies can help a parent make the transition from work to baby comforting (see Chapter 8 for a discussion of Bach flower remedies). Rescue Remedy, an emergency remedy containing five different flowers, not only helps overcome a trauma in an actual emergency (it can help most people stop crying), but is useful when you can't think of the right flower to take.

If you don't think you have the energy to face the many tasks of the evening ahead, take either Olive or Hornbeam. Take Clematis if you feel spacey and unconcentrated. Try Larch if you feel you need additional confidence in dealing with household problems or your child. If you are stewing about something that happened during the day and can't shake it, and if you can associate that feeling as anger, use Holly.

These remedies are for the caregiver, but over the years I have often used them for children. Add a drop or two in some water and apply on the forehead and/or for an infant dilute a drop in some water and place a drop or two under the tongue using an eyedropper. An older child can sip two to four drops in some water or take the preparation under the tongue.

---

children who fall asleep easily but wake up before dawn about 3 or 4 A.M. and can't fall back to sleep until morning.

NIGHTTIME PACIFIER PROBLEMS

"Whenever the pacifier drops out of my baby's mouth, he wakes up from sleep" is a common complaint of young parents. The infant or toddler can be sleeping calmly, yet he cries when he loses his pacifier, so the parent stumbles in, finds the pacifier and replaces it in the child's mouth. When this happens often enough, it contributes to an irregular sleep routine as well as sleep deprivation on the part of the tired parent.

After the age of ten months, children lose the bacteria-fighting antibodies they inherit from their mother, and many pediatricians believe the constant use of pacifiers may cause recurrent ear infections. This is because a pacifier stimulates the flow of saliva, which carries bacteria from the mouth to the throat to the middle ear passages. In fact, Finnish pediatricians did a study showing the relationship of pacifiers and middle ear infections. They recommend that because of the prevalence of ear infections, especially among children in day care, babies should be weaned from their pacifiers by 10 months of age.

The Solution

Gradually decrease the amount of time the child keeps the pacifier in her mouth. This can be accomplished more easily in the daytime when you can distract the child with peek-a-boo and other games. (Experts say good things about the book *Learning Games* by Sparling and Lewis (Warner) because the more than two hundred activities provided are designed to generate social, brain, motor and language development.) With these and other distractions, the baby will need the pacifier less and less. If you also decide to decrease pacifier time during the night, then respond more slowly than usual when the baby cries. Don't go in the minute the baby fusses, but delay your response by five minutes at a time.

You can also give a fussy baby the tissue salt 6c/x Kali Phos. Crush a tablet in a tablespoon of water, and give it to the child in an eye dropper every other hour.

MY BABY WAKES UP EARLY AND DEMANDS TO BE FED FIRST THING

A baby who gets up early every day may be a lark (early-phase sleep pattern) who likes to go to bed early as well. They always feel lively and spirited first thing in the morning. While you can't change the constitution and proclivity of a child who awakens and functions on the early side, you can modify the situation so that it doesn't completely destroy your own sleep cycle.

The Solution

Let's say the baby is getting up at 5 A.M. each morning, but you would like her to get up nearer to 6 or even 7 A.M. Your goal is to change the child's perception of awakening and being fed immediately.

Set up a small schedule on your calendar. This does double duty as it also indicates your progress. Deliberately loiter each morning when your child awakens and delay giving the bottle or breastfeeding the infant first by five minutes. Slowly increase the response time by ten minutes. Within a week or two you will have delayed the time by a half hour. After this first small victory, gradually delay the time more and more until your

Do Nighttime Feedings Lessen Wakenings?

Pediatricians vary in their recommendations of whether or not to fill a wakeful child with some cereal before bedtime. Most think it unwise and usually agree that most babies do not need solid food until six months of age. Then it seems to depend on the child's ability to suck. A test of sucking ability is supplied by pediatrician Dr. William Sears, author of *Nighttime Parenting*. He suggets placing a tiny bit of very ripe mashed banana on the tip of your finger and then on the baby's tongue. If the tongue goes in, the baby's ready to eat solid food. If the tongue comes out, she's not. But even if the baby is ready to eat solid food, Dr. Sears does not recommend feeding cereal before bedtime, because he's found it does not lessen nightwaking.

---

child is sleeping longer and waking up by 6 or 7 A.M. All it requires is patience to reach your goal.

Another technique is to change naptime. Do not let your baby nap as early as he might like, but gradually, in fifteen-minute increments, make the nap later and later until he takes a morning nap about 10 or even 10:30 A.M.

MY BABY DEMANDS TO BE ROCKED TO SLEEP

Rocking a child seems so natural and wonderful; most lullabies refer to every conceivable form of rocking. While there is nothing wrong with holding a baby and rocking her, children often become dependent on this soothing and swaying motion. It only takes a few experiences for an association to be imprinted in the baby's mind. Put yourself in the child's place: "I'm sleepy. I cry. Someone picks me up and rocks me. Great! Then I either sleep until I wake up and cry for someone to rock me again, or I wake up when the rocking stops." For this baby sleeping and rocking form an entwined memory. As desperate parents sometimes learn to their regret, children who are consistently rocked cannot or will not fall asleep on their own. Unless the arrangement is renegotiated, this dependency can sometimes last until the age of four.

A wide group of pediatric sleep specialists advise parents that all children can learn to fall asleep without being rocked on a regular basis. These experts don't say you shouldn't interact with your child in a loving and sweet manner before bedtime. Rather, they stress the need to put children down awake so that they can learn to establish their own methods of drifting off to sleep.

The Solution

Start each new nighttime sleep period with a cozy, warm bath. Sing or murmur lullabies as you envelop the child in a large towel. Parentese—the murmuring of nonsense sounds in a sing-song voice—comes naturally to all parents throughout the world. This is the ideal time for unrestrained, affectionate parentese patter. Infants are fascinated and will understand your tone and be bewitched by your hypnotic reassuring sounds.

After the bath, recite some rhythmic poetry as you dress the baby for bed. After placing him in his crib, read a fictional story or improvise one about your family or the baby's day. Do all this in a quiet sing-song voice. Then begin coaxing her to sleep with something like this: "Time to go to sleep, sweetheart. Baby sleep. Baby sleep. Baby sleeeeepy. Baaby, baaaby is going right to sleep tonight and all nights after this one in her own crib." Murmur lots of such sweet sounds, smile at the baby, pat the baby. Put the baby on his back or side, preferably in a specially designed pillow arrangement. Turn on a cassette of mesmerizing lullabies or one that duplicates white noise effects, the sound of the mother's heart beat or the swish of the in-utero sounds that the baby heard during gestation. If the baby is very young, you might consider placing a loud ticking clock in the room; it will sound a lot like the mother's heartbeat that the baby heard while in the womb. Put one of the baby's thumbs in the opposite fist. (Gripping the thumb is an ancient Asian folk technique to aid sleep. Not only is it comforting, but it will make the child feel as if he is in control.) Tip-toe out of the room.

Since your child's learned expectation is to cry to get someone to rock her to sleep, she will undoubtedly react to being put down by fussing and crying out. Briefly go back into the room. Gently pat her down, and in a low, calm voice reassure, comfort and console the baby, but do not rock her! Again leave the room. You can expect to come and go many times in this same nonjudgmental fashion. However, gradually lengthen the time between each visit. (This also works for naptimes.)

If you are consistent and patient, your child will eventually comprehend this new routine and fall asleep on her own. Make sure you are out of the room (even if only behind the door) when she does fall asleep.

The homeopathic remedy 6c/x Chamomilla is also helpful when coping with children who demand to be rocked to sleep, but be aware that it doesn't satisfy them for long. For infants and toddlers, crush and dissolve one tablet in a tablespoon of water and place it under the child's tongue with an eyedropper.

At-a-Glance Chart of Infant to Toddler Natural Sleep Remedies

For a complete discussion of both homeopathic remedies and tissue salts, see Chapter 7. When administering the homeopathic remedies listed in the following chart, give an infant a half or whole tablet of 3c/x to 12c/x dissolved in a tablespoon of pure spring water or distilled water. For the tissue salts listed in the following chart, give an infant one tablet dissolved in pure spring or distilled water. Give both doses to the infant in an eyedropper or for an older child add to a water bottle. In most instances one dose will be enough to remedy the problem, unless otherwise noted.

Note that throughout the chart the abbreviation H stands for homeopathic remedy and TS stands for tissue salts. Dosage sizes have been abbreviated to read, for example, "6c/x"; however, when buying them, you must ask for either 6c or 6x.

INFANTS TO TODDLERS

HEALTH/SLEEP PROBLEM	NATURAL REMEDIES
GENERAL	• Water therapy: Each night give child warm, relaxing bath. This is also good strategy when child is irritable, restless or crying. Strong bedtime routine is important. • Herbal helps: Sleepless children respond to chamomile herbal tea. • Read Part III, Natural Remedies.
INABILITY TO SLEEP Sleeplessness.	• ½ to 1 tablet H 6c/x Coffea. • If nursing, mother can take adult dose H 6c/x Coffea.
Fussy, has tantrums and cannot get to sleep.	1 tablet TS 6c/x Kali Phos.
Likes to be rocked to sleep.	½ to 1 tablet H 6c/x Pulsatilla.

Infants to toddlers Health/Sleep Problem	Natural Remedies
Won't sleep and has constant need to nurse. (Not only is this exhausting for mother, but it may be beginning of an acquired sleep problem.)	• You must create new associations between food and sleep (rather than weaning). Change nursing schedule: Do not nurse at bedtime, but earlier in evening. Whenever child falls asleep, place in crib. • Be careful child is not taking too much liquid, which disturbs sleep patterns (see below). • Check with pediatrician: If baby is over six months and demonstrates adequate sucking ability, ask if it is time for a prebedtime cereal. • 1 tablet TS 6c/x Calcarea Phos. several times a day for 10 to 14 days. • If nursing mother must drink coffee (she shouldn't), she should take 1 tablet H 6c/x Coffea.
Prone to hiccups just after nursing.	Lay baby on stomach on your lap. If doesn't help, try 1 tablet 6c/x Magnesia Phos.
Awake all night and sleeps only 6 hours during day (sleep pattern continues after first few weeks).	To reverse sleep/wake schedule: Reduce daytime sleep by 10 minutes each day. After weeks of being awakened earlier and earlier, child will consider long daytime sleep a nap and will naturally make nighttime longest sleep period.
Can't sleep because the room is too warm.	• Cool rooms aid sleep, and children's room should have lots of air throughout year. • Make sure child is not dressed too warmly for weather and blankets are not too warm.

Infants to toddlers Health/Sleep Problem	Natural Remedies
	• If room is too warm because of weather or child is ill and you don't want drafts, give ½ to 1 tablet H 6c/x Argentum nit.
Very irritable and can't fall asleep even though very sleepy.	½ to 1 tablet H 6c/x Chamomilla.
Drinking too much liquid, which disrupts sleep patterns.	• Never put infants to sleep with milk bottle or nursing. Besides creating avoidable sleep problem, sugar in milk decays teeth. If bottle is necessary, use water. • Problem most parents have is how to measure infant's hunger. If you think too much liquid is the problem, establish new targets: start by eliminating 1 ounce every or every other evening and lengthen time between feedings. By end of week, aim for 1 ounce before sleep or shorten nursing by a few minutes each evening. Aim for 2 hours between feedings and eventually work up to about 5 hours between feedings.
Hard time falling asleep because of teething problems. Drools a lot.	1 tablet TS 6c/x Nat. Mur.
Can't sleep because of excitement.	1 tablet TS 6c/x Kali Phos.

HEALTH/SLEEP PROBLEM	NATURAL REMEDIES
Can't sleep because of itching or hives.	• 1 tablet TS 6c/x Nat. Phos. • Water therapy: Buy colloidal oatmeal (Aveeno) in drugstore. (If not available, put oatmeal into blender and make powder.) Wet 2 tablespoons, form into paste and apply to itchy parts; when preparing warm bath, add 1 tablespoon or more to bath water. • If nursing, mother should review things she has eaten (spicy foods, for example) that may have caused itching. • If persists, may be a possible food sensitivity to dairy foods, cow's milk and/or wheat.
When child awakens, sleep has not refreshed or restored him.	1 tablet TS 6c/x Nat. Mur.
DURING-SLEEP PROBLEMS Muscles twitch before falling asleep.	1 tablet TS 6c/x Kali Phos.
Twitches during sleep.	1 tablet TS 6c/x Nat. Sulph.
Awakened by gas (flatulence).	• 1 tablet TS 6c/x Nat. Sulph. • Herbs: Add tablespoons of strained tea made with bruised anise, caraway or dill seeds to water bottle. Breastfeeding mothers may drink copious amounts of these herbs to avoid flatulence in child.
Starts (moves suddenly and involuntarily) during sleep.	1 tablet TS 6c/x Nat. Mur.

Infants to Toddlers Health/Sleep Problem	Natural Remedies
Screams during sleep or wakes up screaming.	1 tablet TS 6c/x Kali Phos.
Cries out during sleep.	1 tablet TS 6c/x Calcarea Phos.
Restless sleep	1 tablet TS 6c/x alternately Nat. Phos., Ferrum Phos. and Kali Phos. Check timing in Chap. 8.
Child demands to sleep in parents' bed at night.	May seem easy way out at first, but will lead to acquired sleep problem. Use behavior modification (see text) to put child to sleep awake in own crib.
Child is fearful of dark and demands to sleep in parents' bed.	½ to 1 tablet H 6c/x Pulsatilla 2 or 3 times a day for 10 to 14 days.
Loss of pacifier causes child to awaken.	• Wean child from pacifier slowly during daytime hours. • To overcome fussiness during night, give 1 tablet TS 6c/x Kali Phos.
Teething problems make child irritable and cause moans during sleep. May be difficult to calm child when wakes up.	½ to 1 tablet H 3c/x or 6c/x Chamomilla 1 hour before bedtime and every 30 minutes if child wakes for up to 10 doses.
Pain from teething causes child to toss and turn during sleep. Pain may make child frightened.	½ to 1 tablet H 30c/x Aconite every 30 minutes or more frequently up to ten doses.

Infants to Toddlers Health/Sleep Problem	Natural Remedies
NAPS By 3 to 4 months most babies sleep through night in 5-to-9-hour session and nap 3 or 4 times during day, with one longer session of wakefulness. By 6 months baby should be sleeping about 12 hours at night and take two 1-to-2-hour naps each day. Total sleeptime about 14½ hours.	
Sleepless during night, but can sleep in short naps.	½ to 1 tablet H 6c/x Sulphur every 3 to 4 hours.
Late nap is interfering with getting to bed early. (Child who naps between 4 to 6 P.M. usually can't be put to bed again before 9 or 10 P.M.)	Rearrange pattern of naps as child gets older and can be awake more. Even if child gets very sleepy early in morning, delay nap until 10 or 10:30 A.M. Start by delaying nap by 10 minutes every other day until arrive at desired time. Move afternoon nap to just after lunchtime. Reconditioning takes about 2 weeks.
SLEEPY/OR DROWSY DURING NORMAL AWAKE TIMES Wakes up too late each morning and may be cranky when awakened. (Child is owl with late-phase sleep pattern.)	Follow instructions for Inappropriate Wakefulness below.
Feels and acts sleepy but cannot fall asleep.	½ to 1 tablet H 6c/x Chamomilla every 2 to 3 hours up to 10 doses.
Acts sleepy during time it should be awake and lively, or wakes up tired after a night's sleep.	1 tablet TS 6c/x Nat. Mur.

INFANTS TO TODDLERS

HEALTH/SLEEP PROBLEM	NATURAL REMEDIES
Great drowsiness during normal awake times.	1 tablet TS 6c/x Silica.
Hard to awaken in morning.	1 tablet TS 6c/x Calcarea Phos.
Drowsy in afternoon.	1 tablet TS 6c/x Ferrum Phos.
Drowsiness during day with indigestion.	1 tablet TS 6c/x Nat. Sulph. (Helps with last stages of digestion and disposing of waste materials.)
Drowsy with fever throughout afternoon but can't sleep at night.	1 tablet TS 6c/x Ferrum Phos. every 3 to 4 hours.
INAPPROPRIATE WAKEFULNESS Bedtimes and awakenings do not match, so some children are awake when they should be going to bed or, conversely, may have a problem staying awake until normal bedtime and therefore get up too early in morning.	
Resists going to bed because of anxieties about separating from parents.	½ to 1 tablet H 6c/x Pulsatilla every 1 to 2 hours up to 10 doses.
Gets up too early: early-phase sleep syndrome.	To end self-perpetuating cycle, rearrange .aptimes (see Naps above) and delay your response by 10 minutes when child wakes up. Do this for several days until you reach 5:30 A.M. After that small victory, gradually work toward 6:30 or 7:30 A.M. as desired. Reconditioning takes about 2 weeks.

HEALTH/SLEEP PROBLEM	NATURAL REMEDIES
Gets up too late: late-phase sleep syndrome.	Begin reconditioning program that takes several months' time: Wake child up 10 to 15 minutes earlier than usual for 2 days. Advance time of waking by 5, 10 or 15 minutes every 2 days until you have moved morning wakeup to 1 hour earlier or whatever is desired. Child will be tired, but don't allow additional time for nap. Wake child at same early hour every day, even on the weekends.
WAKEFULNESS Generally wakeful when it is time to sleep.	1 tablet TS 6c/x Kali Phos. and Ferrum Phos., alternating on hour and half hour.
Awake all night, but sleeps 6 hours during day.	Read related section in Inability to Sleep above.
Wide awake and irritable during the first part of the night and wants to be carried around.	½ to 1 tablet H 30c/x Chamomilla. Repeat dose if child awakens from sleep. If chronic condition, follow instructions for chronic situation under homeopathy in Chapter 8.
Sleepy during day but wakeful at night.	1 tablet TS 6c/x Calcarea Sulph.
Hypersensitive to sound.	½ to 1 tablet H 6c/x Coffea 3 times a day for 10 to 14 days.
Light sleeper who reacts to every sound.	½ to 1 tablet H 6c/x Ignatia 3 times a day for 10 to 14 days.

INFANTS TO TODDLERS HEALTH/SLEEP PROBLEM	NATURAL REMEDIES
Sensitive to noise and irritated by every disturbance.	• ½ to 1 tablet H 6c/x Nux Vomica 3 times a day for 10 to 14 days. • Relocate crib in quieter place in house away from household and outside traffic or people noise. • Buy heavy-duty anti-noise drapes or shades for room. • If space is an issue and child is very sensitive to noise, devise a hospital-style ceiling track with curtains that surround crib.
Wants to be carried around.	1 tablet TS 6c/x Kali Phos.
Wants to be fed every hour.	Deliberately stall between feedings by 10 minutes the first 2 days, then gradually increase delay until you are feeding child about every 2½ hours.
Waking up too early in the morning and needs to eat instantly.	Same as Gets Up Too Early under Inappropriate Wakefulness.

MEDICAL AND OTHER SITUATIONS
AIRPLANE FLIGHT

When possible, choose flight that normally coincides with child's sleep routine. Reserve bulkhead seat and bassinet for baby to sleep in. Board early. Reassure baby before and during flight by talking in gentle, soothing voice. Plan to give child bottle of water or preheated milk during both take off and landing; swallowing will help normalize ear pressure. Take along favorite soft toys.

COLIC
- Doubles up with sudden, acute abdominal pain in umbilical area. When severe, often doubled over.
- May have watery diarrhea.
- Angry crying and wants to be held.
- Needs to be held, rocked or walked to get to sleep. Even when colic is conquered, child will need rocking and holding.

- 1 tablet TS 6c/x Magnesia Phos. Discontinue if doesn't work within hour.
- Can alternate 1 tablet TS Magnesia Phos. with ½ to 1 tablet H 6c/x or 12c/x Colocynthis.
- ½ to 1 tablet H 6c/x Chamomilla (also 9c/x, 12c/x, 15c/x, 20c/x doses) every 5 minutes up to 10 doses. Or give few drops 3 times a day. Discontinue if doesn't work (see Chapter 8). 6c/x can also be used anytime child is restless and irritable.
- Chamomile flower tea is very helpful; make sure to use pure flower heads to avoid possible ragweed contamination.
- Make tea of bruised, strained anise, caraway or dill seeds. Add to mother's diet and to child's water bottle.
- Water therapy: Dip a folded cloth into chamomile tea, wring out, apply to baby's abdomen and cover with dry towel until the wet towel gets hot. Repeat.
- Nursing mothers should add yogurt, acidophilus or bifidus capsules to diet.

CONSTIPATION
Inability to evacuate waste materials will make child irritable and sleepless.

Water therapy: Give child tablespoon of pure, filtered water every half hour and before long stools will be soft.

INFANTS TO TODDLERS
HEALTH/SLEEP PROBLEM   NATURAL REMEDIES

CRYING
The sound of crying is disturbing
to parents, so it helps to learn to
distinguish such different sounds
as distress, discomfort, hunger,
anger and fear. Just make sure you
don't act angry; children can easily
feel forsaken or abandoned. Parents can also be too kind and end
up with short-term solutions (like
rocking or taking a child to bed),
which may evolve into long-term
acquired sleeping problems. Eventually even a child who cries a lot
must learn how to settle down and
fall asleep on his own.

- 1 tablet TS 6c/x Kali Phos.
- Water therapy: Father of water
  therapy Sebastian Kneipp advised parents to quickly dip crying children into warm bath and
  immediately envelop them in
  large, warm towels. This works
  for most kids, even for nighttime tantrums. If infant is very
  agitated, place several drops of
  valerian tincture in water or
  apply several drops of the Bach
  flower Rescue Remedy in bath
  or dilute and apply to infant's
  forehead and lips.
- Avoid feeding baby every time
  she cries. Try walking with
  child, outdoors if possible, stroking and singing to distract child.
- See Resources for helpful sleep
  cassettes and crib devices.

Unexpected fit of crying.

- Is infant reacting to something
  new or missing in environment?
  (My newborn always reacted
  with nighttime crying when my
  husband was away for a few
  days!)
- Could it be early evidence of
  sensitivity to milk and lactose
  products or wheat? Are you carefully introducing only one new
  food at a time?
- Maybe this is just an appropriate moment for reassurance.

Excessive flow of tears.   1 tablet TS 6c/x Nat. Mur.

HEALTH/SLEEP PROBLEM	NATURAL REMEDIES
Awakens crying from nightmare and you suspect indigestion.	• 1 tablet TS 6c/x Kali Sulph. or Nat. Sulph. • Water healing for indigestion: Saturate cloth with above dose crushed in warm water, wring out, place on baby's abdomen and massage gently.
DRY THROAT AND EYES	• 1 tablet TS 6c/x. Nat. Mur. • Have child sip pure water.
EXCITED Overexcited and too tired to sleep.	• 1 tablet TS 6c/x Ferrum Phos. and Nat. Phos. used alternately, one on hour, other on half hour. • Water therapy: Quickly dip baby into warm water in basin. Most babies will calm down and fall asleep immediately.
FEVER Fever is nature's sign that body is fighting infection.	• Have child sip lots of cool to cold water, which flushes out infection and reduces fever internally. • Water therapy: Give child cold friction rub (described in Chapter 9). • See author's *The Complete Book of Water Therapy* for more safe ways to reduce fever.
Feverish congestion makes child feel like sleeping in afternoon but cannot sleep at night.	• Child needs water. • 1 tablet TS 6c/x Ferrum Phos. every 3 to 4 hours. As fever subsides, lengthen time between doses.
Can't fall or stay asleep because of fever; tosses and turns in crib.	½ to 1 tablet H 6c/x Aconitum 3 times during day.

INFANTS TO TODDLERS HEALTH/SLEEP PROBLEM	NATURAL REMEDIES
FUSSY Cross and grumpy, has temper tantrums and can't sleep.	• 1 tablet TS 6c/x Kali Phos. • Warm bath works miracles on grumpy children.
GAS Extreme flatulence and gas makes infant very uncomfortable; child cries and screams in pain.	• Crush several fennel, anise or dill seeds to release volatile oils, steep in cup of boiling water, strain out seeds, cool tea and add to water bottle. • Nursing mothers can add these teas to their diets to avoid flatulence in baby. • Also read Colic.
ILL-TEMPERED Before or while going to sleep.	1 tablet TS 6c/x Kali Phos.
JERKING LIMBS DURING SLEEP	1 tablet TS 6c/x Silica and Nat. Sulph. alternately, 3 times a day up to 10 days.
NURSING Since every cry is not a cry of hunger, it is essential to endure and tolerate some crying. Ask yourself if it's really a cry of hunger. Learn to interpret and follow your infant's signals.	• Read Won't Sleep and Has Constant Need to Nurse under Inability to Sleep above. • Rather than nurse too often, develop alternate strategies: give baby a warm bath, stroke or sing to baby, listen to music together, take baby for walk in stroller or ride in car.
TEETHING PROBLEMS	• Massage infant's gums with fingertips, whiskey or mixture of one drop of clove oil (strong anesthetic) added to two tablespoons of sunflower or safflower oil. Be sure not to overdo clove oil.

INFANTS TO TODDLERS
HEALTH/SLEEP PROBLEM   NATURAL REMEDIES

	• Frozen items: In separate plastic bags, freeze clean washcloths for child to suck on when uncomfortable. Make your own iced teething ring: Freeze clean, chewable, holdable rubber toy to suck on. • Weleda carries Orris root to suck on (see Resources). • Mother can lessen and/or avoid late teething in child by taking 5 tablets TS 6c/x Calcarea Phos. 3 times a day in last 2 months of pregnancy.
Irritable, angry child may moan during sleep; won't calm down after waking up.	½ to 1 tablet H 6c/x Chamomilla 1 hour before bedtime and every 30 minutes if child awakens up to 6 doses.
Hard time falling asleep; drools a lot even during sleep.	1 tablet TS 6c/x Nat. Mur.
Cough from teething.	1 tablet TS 6c/x Calcarea Phos.
Diarrhea (undigested slimy, green stools) and acute colic while teething.	1 tablet TS 6c/x Calcarea Phos.
Acute pain from sudden teething. Scared by pain, baby tosses and turns during sleep.	½ to 1 tablet H 30c/x Aconite every 30 minutes or if the pain persists more frequently up to 10 doses.
Spasmodic colic with diarrhea.	1 tablet TS 6c/x Magnesia Phos. in hot water every 15 minutes.
Restless and irritable, swollen gums, flushed face, hot with fever.	1 tablet TS 6c/x Ferrum Phos. every hour up to 10 doses.

INFANTS TO TODDLERS HEALTH/SLEEP PROBLEM	NATURAL REMEDIES
TESTY AND IRRITABLE Peevish and fretful during day before going to sleep or when coming out of sleep.	1 tablet TS 6c/x Calcarea Phos. Repeat if child awakens from sleep.
THRUSH Yeast infection in mouth or on scalp.	• 1 tablet TS 6c/x Kali Mur. every 1 to 2 hours. • Add 1 teaspoon liquid bifidus (soy or milk based) to water or milk bottle. • Rub child's head and massage skin with pure flaxseed oil (always refrigerate). Warm oil in hands before massage.
VOMITING Vomits sour curdled milk.	• 1 tablet TS 6c/x Calcarea Phos. and Nat. Phos. alternate one on hour, other on half hour. • Water therapy: Dip dish towel into three tablespoons of apple cider vinegar and a 1/4 cup of water, wring out, place on child's abdomen and cover with dry cloth. Renew as soon as towel gets hot. • Have child sip bruised fennel seed tea.
YAWNING Spasmodic. Excessive.	1 tablet TS 6c/x Silica. 1/2 to 1 tablet H 6c/x Ignatia 3 times a day for 10 days.

6

Dealing with Childhood Sleep Problems

While infants sleep as long as sixteen, even seventeen hours a day, sleeptime lessens with age. By two years old the average child naps and sleeps about twelve to fourteen hours. Most children from four to twelve need about ten or eleven hours of sleep. Children often establish their mode of sleep- and waketime early in life. Some people seem to be born larks. The inventor Thomas Edison only slept four hours at night and took a series of extremely short catnaps during the day. Napoleon was another lark. "Six hours for a man, seven hours for a woman, eight hours for a fool," he advised subordinates about sleep. Some people seem to naturally need less sleep than others.

Fortunately, most children settle into a good night's sleep by age three months. However, if good sleep habits aren't settled by a year and a half, watch out. At eighteen months children discover their own personal power mode. Their sense of self tells them that they can command, so they can tell their parents what they want and get it. That starts the tug of power between child and parent. If a parent doesn't set the tone early and if the child isn't made to realize the parent is gently in control, a willful child will establish a warring beachhead. Fortunately, most children are amenable to gentle and consistent power arrangements. (For an illuminating discussion of the correlation between sleep and a child's temperament, see the Appendix.)

Some Childhood Sleep Disturbances

The major source of sleep problems in school children is adjusting to new situations in daycare or school. Having a new teacher or aide, dealing with a difficult homework assignment, facing a big test, competing in a spelling

Sleep Stages of Children from 3 to 18

AGE	TIME FRAME	MISC. FACTS
THREE YEARS TO PREADOLESCENCE	11 hours	• Abnormal behavior: Confusion, thrashing, possible bedwetting, sleepwalking, night terrors, in which child shows waking and sleeping traits at same time. • Can take child to urinate and will return to sleep immediately since arousal is only partial.
PREADOLESCENTS	10 hours	
ELEVEN TO FOURTEEN YEARS	Starts at 9½ hours, goes down to 9 hours.	
FIFTEEN TO EIGHTEEN YEARS	Can sleep 8-plus hours a day, but normally gets only 7-8 hours or less, which is insufficient.	

When to Expect Possible Sleep Problems

- The family is on a trip.
- If the daily routine is disrupted: daytime visitors or overnight or long-term visitors unsettle the daily schedule.
- When a sister or brother is born.
- When the child or a parent is ill.
- Moving from one home to another.
- A new babysitting or daycare arrangement.

bee or having a run-in with another child might all disrupt your child's usual sleep pattern. Other sources of problems may be changes in the family routine, times when the parents are ill or away on business and if there are long-term guests. A sudden case of crankiness and/or irritability might also arise because the child simply needs more sleep. Try sending the youngster to bed a half hour to an hour earlier for a day or two.

However, some sleep problems run deeper and are more difficult to handle. Nightmares, sleep walking, night terrors, sleep apnea and attention-deficit disorders all pose unique but ultimately manageable sleep problems.

NIGHTMARES

When a child awakens from a frightening dream in the dark, the darkness may invoke some of the primitive fear of our ancient cave-dwelling ancestors. Even though dreaming has been the subject of many studies and much speculation, no one yet knows for sure where dreams, good and bad, come from. Maybe bad dreams stem from an inability to sort out new experiences and new rules that confound the child during the day. Whatever the cause, many children between the ages of three and six wake up crying in the night and report scary dreams of being chased by monsters. It's best to soothe and reassure the child and encourage him to get right back to sleep, surrounded and protected by his favorite toys.

There are ways you can prepare for such episodes:

- Check the at-a-glance chart at the end of this chapter for natural remedies that help with nightmares. Be sure to have them on hand so you can deal with the problem whenever it arises.
- Use an unobtrusive lamp that gradually dims to darkness in the child's room. The gradual dimming of the light reassures a frightened child that there are no monsters, aliens or robots in the room.
- The next day, talk to the child about the bad dream. Gently probe for one or more possible reasons for the child's unease. Is it based on an event the day before? Is someone teasing or scaring the child? Does the disturbance stem from a frightening TV cartoon or video? Have you or your daycare center recently cut out a nap after lunch? Perhaps your child is just overtired, in which case you can see that the nap is reinstituted for a while. (See other suggestions for talking about nightmares in the scenarios section of this chapter.)

SLEEPWALKING

While most episodes of sleepwalking are merely sitting-up-in-bed incidents, some children, most frequently between the ages of four and eight, do walk in their sleep. Sleepwalking occurs in the first several hours of the night during the deepest period of sleep. Dr. Richard Ferber, director of the Center for Pediatric Sleep Disorders, Children's Hospital, Boston, says the children who sleepwalk have "an incomplete waking from deep nondreaming sleep." In other words, sleepwalking is a partial waking. Apparently children who sleepwalk and who have night terrors (see below) do not make an adequate brain wave transition from one stage of sleep to waking. So the child has a "simultaneous functioning of both the child's waking and deep sleep system," says Dr. Ferber. "Both processes seem to be going on together. The child is both asleep and awake at the same time." During sleepwalking and night terrors the "child's eyes are open, but she has no awareness of what is going on around her. Children may stare at you, mumble phrases, walk down stairs, open doors and leave the house," says Dr. Ferber. During such an incident, in the child's disorientation and confusion, he may inappropriately urinate in the wrong place—sometimes in a closet. Ferber suggests you try to gently guide the sleepwalking child to urinate in the bathroom and proceed back to bed.

You can take the following steps to ensure that the child doesn't hurt himself during sleepwalking:

- Unclutter the child's room.
- If the child is sleeping in a bunk bed, it's safer to have him sleep on the lower bunk.
- Put locks on the windows in the child's room.
- Put a bell on the child's door to wake you if the child leaves her room.
- Consider putting a gate at the top of the stairs, or take all objects off the stairs and leave the light on in the stairwell.
- Put chain locks high enough on all outside doors so that the child cannot get out of the house by merely opening a door.

NIGHT TERRORS

Night terrors, which usually occur during the first hours of a child's sleep, are quite common in children between the ages of four and twelve. They have been characterized as "intense arousal" by famed pediatric sleep expert Dr. Richard Ferber and co-authors in *Principles and Practices of Sleep Medi-*

cine in Children. (Read about sleepwalking above, which is another type of partial arousal.)

In a night terror, as against a nightmare when a child awakens from a bad dream, the child is actually not awake, although she is sitting up flushed, disoriented, sweating and screaming blood-curdling shrieks, with her eyes wide open and bulging. "The facial expression is one of intense fear," writes Dr. Ferber. "In a full-blown episode, a youngster may jump out of bed and run blindly, as if away from some unseen threat. This may be very dangerous, and injury during this frenzied activity is quite possible. The youngster may knock over furniture or even break windows. Anyone attempting to intervene may also be injured."

If such an incident occurs, take the following steps:

- Reassure your child quietly.
- Do not ask questions about the "dream." Children do not remember such incidents in the morning.
- Expect your attempts to comfort your child to go unheeded.
- Make common-sense security arrangements about open windows, stairwells and doors.
- Usually such terrors gradually disappear as the child grows up.

However, according to Dr. Ferber, if your child is beyond six years of age and night terrors persist, appear for the first time or recur, there may be a minor psychological problem that you need to deal with. (See Resources at the end of the book for a national organization to help you locate a sleep disorder clinic and a pediatric sleep specialist in your area.)

"In milder forms, these disorders of arousal are quite common, especially in children, and *require no intervention* or *only for safety*. . . . In some children, the arousals may be frequent, very disruptive, or dangerous, and pharmacologic treatment or relaxation and mental imagery training is often very effective," writes Dr. Ferber.

There are a number of safety precautions you can take:

- Safety-proof the windows, stairs and door as you would for sleepwalking.
- Make sure the child isn't too tired during the day. Daytime and nighttime routines should be quiet and consistent.
- If the child is young and a daytime nap has recently been omitted, reschedule one for the late morning or just after lunch. (Also read about naps in the At-a-Glance Chart at the end of the chapter.)
- Usually night terrors occur within the first hours of the child's sleep when the parents are still awake. If the incidents continue, note the time they start. Many parents have found they can control the episodes and avoid future ones if they wake the child up fifteen minutes

before the anticipated time, stay with the child for five to ten minutes and then quietly persuade him to go back to sleep. Continue to do this until the night terrors stop. You can establish the same procedure if the night terrors start once again.

SLEEP APNEA

Apnea means the absence of breathing. When this temporary stoppage of breathing occurs during sleep, it can lead to many physical and mental problems, including behavioral upsets, tiredness and forgetfulness. If your child snores loudly and sometimes appears to be struggling to breathe during sleep, complains of morning headaches and has frequent infections of the nasal passages, discuss these problems with your pediatrician.

The most frequent causes of sleep apnea in children are enlarged tonsils or adenoids; the child is too heavy or obese for his age; or teeth, chin or other facial problems exist that will need the attention of a dentist and/or an ear, nose and throat specialist. Once this condition is diagnosed, you may also want to consult a specialist at a local sleep disorders center. These centers are geared to deal successfully with adult sleep apnea and have recently evidenced interest in treating this condition in children.

ATTENTION-DEFICIT DISORDER

Children with attention-deficit disorder tend to be hard to get to bed. Since they get to bed later than they should, they end up sleeping less than other children their age. This means they end up with a sleep deficit. Getting more sleep, even a half hour more each night, can help this type of child focus better the next day. Dr. Ronald E. Dahl, associate professor of psychiatry and pediatrics at the University of Pittsburgh, School of Medicine, suggests that parents work out and stick to an agreed-on sleep routine that can include rewards for going to sleep on time. Dr. Dahl points out that we don't know the consequences of continued sleep deprivation in children, but animal studies show that the immature and growing brain thrives on sleep.

Some natural remedies to help a child with attention-deficit disorder include:

- Give relaxing teas such as catnip and chamomile.
- To keep the child calm and relaxed, add valerian tincture or chamomile tea to the child's bathwater.

- After a long relaxing bath before bed, massage the child, especially his feet and spine, with aromatic oil such as coconut or almond. You can also use olive oil. Or you can add one drop of essential oils, such as chamomile, lavender and rosemary, to two tablespoons of massage oil.

Helpful Sleep Scenarios and Solutions for Children

The following strategies and scenarios are designed to help solve the most prevalent childhood sleep problems. Each includes a parental approach and dialogue as well as proven step-by-step training concepts (also known as behavior modification). Your success with the scenarios depends on your patience, persistence and determination to turn the problem around. Though these techniques have proven effective for most parents and children, nothing is foolproof. If you find something doesn't work or isn't suited to your child's personality, be creative and revamp the scenario. Follow your child's lead and your own instincts and good judgment. Also check the At-a-Glance Chart at the end of the chapter for many homeopathic remedies, water therapies and other natural cures for the following and other problems. (You may also want to read Part III, Natural Sleep Remedies, at the same time.)

MY CHILD DEMANDS TO BE ROCKED TO SLEEP

You can use the same technique for an older child who needs to be rocked or held while going to sleep as for an infant. Only now you can add to the process by giving the child a new stuffed animal and telling her a personalized going-to-bed-on-her-own bedtime story. An older child will be intrigued and fascinated by a personalized story that contains her name and creative facts about her life. As with all bedtime scenarios the element of time is important. Make sure the child knows, perhaps as early as her bath, that something very special will happen that night.

The Solution
Your story can go like this: "Tonight Abigail dearest is going to fall asleep in her bed without being rocked. And tonight—this is a special night—Mommy and Daddy are giving Abigail a new special friend to take to bed

with her. [At this point give the child the new toy.] "This cute little bear [lion, doll] named Sleepy will go to bed with you tonight and all other nights after this, too. Sleepy is going to protect you during the night. Sleepy can sleep next to you or you can hold her. And tonight you are going to sleep this way." [Take one of the child's thumbs and place it in the fist of her other hand.]

If you know the child is having great difficulty with separation, especially if the child is slightly older and has often crept into bed with you, consider the homeopathic remedy Pulsatilla that is also successful for children who need to be rocked. Crush one pill of 3c/x or 6c/x in a tablespoon of water and add to water or milk or have the older child dissolve one tablet under the tongue. (For a thorough discussion of tissue salts see Chapter 8. Note that you can buy them in *either* 3c or 3x sizes, which are abbreviated here as 3c/x.)

MY CHILD PERSISTS IN GETTING OUT OF BED TO PROTEST THE NEW ROUTINE

Firmly and gently tell the child the rules: "This is under your control. If you get out of bed, I will have to close the door. It is your choice." Most children will test this rule at least once. If the child gets out of bed again, close the door for one minute. You can talk reassuringly from behind the closed door. Don't lock the door, but hold on to it so that the child can't open it. This shows the child that having the door open is under her control. If she gets out of bed, the door gets closed. You can use a gate if you want, instead of a door, but stay out of sight when the gate is closed.

If this becomes a contest of wills and the child persists in getting out of bed, increase the time the door is closed from one minute to three minutes and then to five minutes. Let five minutes be the maximum for the first night. It's important for the parent to remember that you are doing this to reinforce a needed concept. This is not a new form of punishment. (It may be appropriate to read the connection between sleep and temperament in the Appendix, if you haven't already.)

On the second night, follow the same scenario of bath, personalized story, giving the child the new stuffed toy and firmly putting the child into her bed. If the child gets out of bed, explain the rules once again: "Sweetheart, if you get out of bed, I will have to close the door. This is your decision. The door is under your control. You have to stay in bed!" If she gets out of her crib again and yet again, close the door for two minutes and work up to five as you did the first night. Keep increasing the time of the door closure as she persists. This is a gradually learned new routine, but it will work over time—you just have to be patient and persistent.

If the child is also getting out of bed during naptime and an hour has elapsed, tell the child naptime is over and go about the normal business of the day.

MY CHILD INSISTS ON SLEEPING IN OUR BED EVERY NIGHT

Some people really enjoy having a child sleep with them every night. California pediatrician Dr. William Sears makes a strong point for this bonding and interaction in his book *Nighttime Parenting*. He advises parents to have the baby sleep in the bed or on a mattress or crib rolled adjacent to the parental bed.

On the other hand, Dr. Richard Ferber in his masterful book, *Solve Your Child's Sleep Problems*, explains the repercussions of a child sleeping each night in his parent's bed. The consequences are several: a child who continuously creeps into the parents' bed doesn't undergo an absolutely needed experience—the learned response of going to sleep on his own. This sleeping arrangement may also create scarring emotional problems. A child who climbs into bed instinctively knows that he is interfering with his Mom and Dad's sleep and becomes subliminally aware, especially if he is sleeping between the two parents, that he has a strange, unknown power that he doesn't know how to cope with. So, ultimately, despite the bonding and the generosity involved in letting a child sleep with adults, this sleeping arrangement prevents a child from achieving the psychological separation he must acquire for later life.

For the above reasons, as well as the achievement of parental privacy, many pediatric researchers recommend weaning the child from his attachment to the parents' bed and teaching the child to fall asleep on his own. Children who reach these two new goals are always grateful for the new guidelines.

The Solution

I met a young lawyer socially, and when he discovered I was writing a book on sleep, he mentioned his sleep concerns about his two-year-old son Robert. It was obvious that the father was crazy about his son. He asked what I thought about the boy coming into the parents' bed each night. I told him the possible advantages, the potential long-range disadvantages and my own feeling about the intrusion into personal nightly privacy. He asked if I had any good ideas about changing the situation. I worked out the following scenario, and a few weeks later the father called and chortled, "It's unbelievable how well your story is working!"

The two parents have to agree on the goal that it is in the best interest of the child and the family to change the situation. As in the scenario to end a child being rocked to sleep every night, you want to interest and excite your child about sleeping in his own crib.

First, buy a cute stuffed animal and call it "Sleepyhead." Keep Sleepyhead wrapped and out of the way until you need it. Also, buy a big business calendar. Pick out a date some two to three weeks ahead and circle it on the calendar. While it isn't necessary, it may be useful if the date has some real or imaginary significance. It also helps if the date is on a weekend so that the father can participate in the changeover. It is good for the parents to take turns telling the story to the child each night; it may help to decide on some of the details of the story so you can alternate easily. Note that it is better not to ask a sitter to do the scenario.

If the child is old enough to change from a crib to a youth bed, purchase the bed with delivery timed to coincide with the target date. If you choose to buy a bed, incorporate it in your bedtime story for the next few weeks.

Use the following story as a baseline—change it, alter it, embellish it. Let your imagination run wild. As you go along, or from the very beginning, add personal details from your child's life. You can add details about your work life (where, when and how you work). You can add details about grandparents and other relatives and how much they love your precious child. Include their names, where they live and if they, or their parents or grandparents, came from another country. Depending on your timeframe, you can add the names of caregivers and neighbors. You can add personal adventures and triumphs of the child as the weeks unfold. In other words, feel free to completely personalize the scenario and make it your very own.

With the calendar marked, the stuffed toy available and any other details of your story's surprise worked out, tell your child just before bedtime that you have a special story to tell. Show your child the calendar and the circled date. The scenario runs like this:

The Script

Something special is going to happen to a child named Robert. Robert is just two years old, yet he can recognize George Washington. So guess what? On Washington's Birthday on February 22—see the date circled on this calendar? That date is three weeks from tonight. On that date, Robert is going to do something new and special.

This boy named Robert is _____ inches high, has _____ hair and _____ eyes. Robert is a great kid, and his parents love him very much. On February 22, Robert is going to get a special present. He is getting this present because he is so grown up for his age.

Who is this boy Robert? Where does he live? He lives at _____ in the county of _____ in the (township, village, city) _____ in the state of _____ in the United States of America. Robert is exactly _____ (months or years) old. Robert's parents _____ and _____ have a telephone and the number is _____.

Robert goes to a playgroup that meets in different houses (or day-care) _____ (days of the week). Robert likes to play with the following kids: _____, _____, _____ and _____. Robert likes to play with toys like _____ , _____ and _____. Robert likes to look at books, and he likes to have stories told to him just before he goes to sleep.

This is the story Robert will hear every night until February 22, the date circled on the calendar. The reason Robert is getting a special present is because he is such a grown-up boy that he deserves to have a special present. So what is the present? Robert will get a new stuffed toy named Sleepyhead. (Optional: Robert will get a second present: his own junior bed.)

This is happening to Robert because he is going to be two years old (whatever age) and on this date (point to circled date), Robert (loud whisper) will sleep in his own bed! Robert will no longer sleep in his parents' bed because he is so grown up and he is getting a new toy named Sleepyhead to sleep with (and he is also getting his own bed).

When Robert sleeps in his crib (or his own bed) with Sleepyhead, Robert will feel safe and cozy, safe and comfy, safe and loved. And what will happen after that date? Every night thereafter, when it is time to fall asleep, Robert will settle down quickly, and magic of magic, he will fall asleep fast! So fast that Robert will become known as the fastest sleeper on _____ street in _____ county in _____ state!

And magic of magic, the crib (or new bed) that Robert is going to sleep in is so very special that Robert (whisper) will sleep right through the night from then on!

And this crib (or new bed) is so very special that even if Robert wakes up sometimes in the night to check his pillow or his blanket, he will always know he is safe. Robert will always know that he is protected. Robert will always go right back to sleep.

Then on the target date, give your child the wrapped gift of Sleepyhead as promised. If the youth or junior bed is also planned, have the bed set up in the room that day. If you plan to have the child visiting somewhere while it is set up, the new bed can come as an additional surprise.

WHAT IF THE STORY DOESN'T WORK
AND THE CHILD GETS OUT OF HIS BED
AND STILL COMES TO YOUR BED?

Don't be too disappointed; this can happen. You may have to invest another two weeks in training your child.

The Solution

If the child pops up at the side of your bed, be firm and patient. Say, "No, dear, remember the story we told you that you were going to sleep in your own crib (or new bed) from now on." Take the child by the hand, and reluctant or not, put him back in his crib (or bed). Then, tell the child, "If you don't stay in bed, I'll have to close the door." Then follow the procedure described above for a child who persists in getting out of bed. This is a very effective technique and usually works within two weeks.

If the child is unusually anxious and continues his behavior, do not agree to lie in your bed or his bed with him, but agree to sit in a chair near the bed. If he gets out of bed, then begin the door closing technique, showing him that the door is under his command. Keep focused on your goal of having the child fall asleep on his own in his own bed. During the next two weeks, gradually move your chair farther and farther away from his bed and nearer the door. At the last stage park your chair just outside his bedroom.

Should your child wake up and start crying but not get out of bed, just tarry a bit until you answer him and keep up the delaying tactics. Crying is always alarming, even irritating to a parent, but your tarrying, gentleness and firmness in the new rule will make this a transient episode.

If your child is so anxious that he cries until he throws up, don't act alarmed or as if you have to acknowledge the act of vomiting. Go into the bedroom, and quietly and gently without judgment or anger, change the bedding and his pajamas. Then leave the room again saying, "Go to sleep, sweetheart. Mommy and Daddy are in the next room. You are safe and comfy, safe and cozy, safe and loved. Now go back to sleep. We'll see you in the morning."

MY CHILD WAKES UP DURING THE NIGHT

Like all people, each child comes with his own internal biological clock, called a "circadian cycle." The clock makes the child aware of sleep, eating and rest signals. The clues for these needs come from changes in temperature and the flow of body hormones as the circadian rhythm is reset each day.

The Solution

If a child's sleep cycle becomes erratic, it can be modified and reset by increasing or decreasing the times of sleeping, awakening, resting and eating. In all cases take the cues from the child as you deliberately restructure the times of sleep and wakefulness in half-hour increments.

Some children awaken on a regular schedule. If your child awakens between midnight and 3 or 4 A.M., use the homeopathic remedy 6c/x Arsenicum, and feed one tablet to the child every 3 to 4 hours as long as the behavior persists, but no longer than ten days. Then discontinue the remedy. (For a thorough discussion of tissue salts see Chapter 8. Note that you can buy them in *either* 3c or 3x sizes, which are abbreviated here as 3c/x.)

For a child who goes to sleep easily but awakens about 3 or 4 A.M. and insists on staying awake for the rest of the night, but then falls asleep when he's supposed to be getting up, use one tablet of homeopathic 3c/x or 6c/x Nux Vomica. This remedy is especially valuable for children who are irritated by noise and generally tend to be worried, anxious or irritable.

MY CHILD WAKES UP TOO EARLY IN THE MORNING

If you have a lark (early-phase sleep problem) in your family, you can still train the child to conform more readily to the entire family's schedule.

The Solution

Try keeping early morning light from coming into the child's room with heavy shades or opaque curtains. Prevent traffic or even household noise from awakening the child by putting a screen around the bed and/or placing a white noise machine in the room to override outside noises.

Deliberately loiter each morning when you respond to your child's awakening, first by five minutes, then by ten minutes. Within a week or two you will have delayed the time by a half hour. Gradually delay the time more and more until your child is sleeping longer and waking up by 6 or 7 A.M. If your child is older, encourage her to go to the bathroom on her own and then play with her toys in bed until Mommy and Daddy get up. Another technique is to change the child's naptime. Do not let the child nap in the morning, but put her down right after lunch. All the training process requires is patience and ingenuity in reaching your goal.

MY CHILD WAKES UP TOO LATE IN THE MORNING

The need and urge to sleep late in the day (late-phase sleep pattern) can start in infancy and continue through life. Owls have a hard time falling asleep at normal bedtimes but like to stay up late and then will go to bed willingly. An owl feels good if allowed to sleep as long as she likes, but will be cranky if awakened too early. Later in life this may make going to school or work an ordeal.

The Solution

This reconditioning is imperative for an owl in a morning playgroup, daycare or school since the child will have trouble getting up in the morning. Fortunately, this program follows the child's own proclivities for going to sleep late and is easy for the child to tolerate. Just remember not to start this reconditioning program during school, but wait for a vacation period.

If the child is waking up at 9:30 A.M. on the first day, wake him up at 9:25 A.M. the next two days in a row. Every two days thereafter wake him up five, ten or fifteen minutes earlier until you reach the time needed for family or school activity.

During this time the child will be slightly sleepy during the day. Most young owls want to add extra sleeptime to their nap. Don't allow this. Both young and somewhat older owls will soon be expressing an interest in going to sleep slightly earlier than usual. Once you reach an adequate level of sleep and a good schedule, keep to that schedule, and absolutely don't vary it on weekends; otherwise you will break the hard-earned new cycle! Consider this routine accomplished when your child wakes on his own at a time that is suitable for his and the family's schedule.

MY CHILD'S PROBLEM WITH A CHILD IN DAYCARE OR A PROBLEM WITH A SIBLING IS INTERFERING WITH SLEEP

A child who has a constant problem with another child in daycare or with a sibling may need the restorative homeopathic remedy 6c/x Nux Vomica. Children who do well with this remedy are those who worry a lot and seem anxious about school and their schoolmates. Have the child take one tablet three times each day at intervals of two to three hours for at least a week and up to two weeks.

WHEN DAYTIME FEARS SHOW UP BEFORE BEDTIME

Many children act out their daytime worries just as they are going to sleep. One common worry that must be addressed by parents and caregivers is children's fears about separation. Many children have deeply rooted fears of abandonment and will indicate them at every separation during the day and often before going to sleep.

The Solution

All children need a calm and predictable routine for sleep, but children who indicate concern about separation particularly need a carefully orchestrated, routinized schedule for their dinner and the time prior to sleep as well as constant reassurance until they get over this anxiety. Make sure that the child does not watch anxiety-provoking or scary television or videos. Carefully pick bedtime stories to avoid frightening situations and concentrate on those that reinforce trust and the feeling of safety. Ask the librarian to recommend stories about children who have had bad dreams and resolved their worries. Play games where the themes are safety and trust. Repeat some funny, easy phrase like "you are as safe and snug as a bug in a rug" every night as you put the child to sleep. If your child is old enough, use techniques for redreaming nightmares and creative dreaming described in Chapter 10.

Early homeopaths discovered that 6c/x or 9c/x Pulsatilla was the perfect help for children who fear separation and abandonment from their parents. This is also used for the child who likes to be rocked before sleep, often climbs into his parents' bed at night, has a constant fear of being alone in the dark and may have nightmares about his parents leaving him. Give the child one tablet every three to four hours as necessary up to ten doses.

DEALING WITH NIGHTMARES

Children find all kinds of reasons to delay going to sleep, and a common one is to avoid recurring nightmares. Children, particularly those with fear of separation, often express their anxieties through nightmares that awaken them. Once awakened, they may have a hard time falling asleep again.

The Solution

As often as possible reassure the child that she will be safe during the day and nighttime. Be matter of fact about the nightmare. Stay with the child for a little while, comfort her and tell her you'll talk about it in the morning.

Talk about the nightmare during the day. Ask her, "What do you remember about that dream you had last night?" As the child unravels the dream, ask specific questions about it. "Did it frighten you? Why do you suppose it scared you?" Try to find out what is making your child anxious and afraid. Bringing out all the details of the frightening experience washes away some of the negative energy of the dream. Think of phrases to say that will reassure the child such as, "Boy, that was some dream! But I never heard of anything like that ever happening in the daytime!" Or something like, "You know, I remember having scary dreams when I was a kid, but I got over it." Or maybe, "You know, anytime something scary happens to you, I want you to come to me and we'll talk it over."

If the child is older, you could try a more direct approach: "Do you suppose you are worrying about something special now, and it came out in your dream? I'm wondering if you are worried about (mention any of the changes that have come up in her life recently, such as meeting new kids at school? Having a new baby sitter? The fight you had with your brother? The next show-and-tell in school?)."

Once your child realizes that her parents understand her fears and that they aren't unreasonable or dumb, she'll feel a lot better and safer. If the nightmares persist, you can find books about dreams and nightmares at the library to read to your child. Or find an old stuffed animal friend or buy a new one that the child can take to bed for comfort. Include the toy in your bedtime stories, and tuck the toy in when you tuck in your youngster. If the child is afraid of the dark, install a small night light, and keep the bedroom door slightly ajar.

ANTI-NIGHTMARE HERBS: Make teas out of any of the following excellent sedative and anti-nightmare herbs:

- German chamomile. One outstanding herbalist from the past considered this "the cure par excellence for nightmares."
- Catnip is the herb traditionally used throughout Great Britain and all through Appalachia for children who had nightmares.
- The following are also excellent sleep-inducing and anti-nightmare herbal teas: marjoram, Melissa (lemon balm), mignonette, thyme or violets.

HOMEOPATHIC REMEDIES:
(For a thorough discussion of homeopathic remedies see Chapter 8. Note that you can by them in *either* 3c or 3x sizes, which are abbreviated here as 3c/x.)

- For children who are agitated before bedtime or who normally awaken from sleep with scary dreams, use homeopathic 3c/x or 6c/x Argentum

Nit. Give a young child one tablet every two to three hours for about a week. For an older child, give two tablets every two to three hours for a week.

- For children who are prone to awaken frequently during the night in a state of terror and who may also be seeing ghosts or animals, use one tablet of homeopathic 3c/x or 6c/x Stramonium for about a week to ten days.
- For emotional children who have frightful dreams at night and who also yawn and stretch a lot during the day, use homeopathic 6c/x Staphysagria. Just before bed, give one tablet and repeat if the child awakens.
- There are two other homeopathic remedies for children who have chronic sleep-disturbing events. Since these are more serious problems, you may want to take your child to a pediatric homeopath for evaluation.

BATHS: Have the child take long, warm soaks. Add a half cup of sleep-inducing herbal teas or two to three drops of chamomile, lavender, pine, sage or thyme essential oils to the bath.

MASSAGE: Use sleep-help nerve-pressure massage on the feet. Starting with the toes, massage the sole, heel, sides, ankle and top of each foot.

DEALING WITH SLEEP DISTURBANCES WHEN SOME BELOVED PERSON DIES

When someone close to a family dies, it deeply affects most children and will often be reflected in sleep problems. The absence of a beloved parent, aunt or uncle, grandparent, sibling or even a neighbor strikes at the very center of a child's need for safety and trust in adults. Therapists have known for a long time that it is best to bring all sense of loss, grief and fear felt by individual members of the family out in the open at such a time. This prevents unresolved fears from festering.

Lying about death bewilders and frightens a child. I have two adult friends who each lost a parent when they were two and four years of age, respectively. In each case those around them chose to ignore the situation as if it didn't happen, and this left deep wounds in each child.

Another situation that frightens many children is being forced to look at their beloved parent, grandparent or sibling in an open coffin. One famous case study that led to terrible lifelong apprehension and dissociation problems resulted from being forced to touch the dead person.

The Solution

It is important for parents or significant caregivers to be honest about their own grief and share it with the child. The library has many good books on death and dying that can be read to the child.

There is an excellent homeopathic remedy for grief. (I can verify from a recent family death how invaluable it is for adults, too.) Homeopathic 6c/x Ignatia is indicated when anyone is confronted with any deep emotional upset and when and if sleep is disturbed after an emotional upset. Often a child who needs Ignatia will yawn a lot. The dose can be repeated every three to four hours for a day or so, depending on the symptoms. For an acute situation, follow the instructions in the homeopathy section in Chapter 8.

NAPTIME PROBLEMS

In the first two years, napping is essential for total sleep. Yet, sometimes too few, too many or too-late-in-the-day naps greatly interfere with the child's functioning and ability to sleep at night. Note that by the child's second year, she will give up most of her naps. Here are solutions to some typical nap problems.

Child Insists on Taking Too Many Naps

You don't want the child to take too many naps, as it will affect her ability to get to sleep at a normal bedtime. What you need to do is eliminate part or all of the daytime naps so that the child on her own will compensate and sleep more easily and for a longer time at night. You have several choices. One is to go cold turkey and just skip the morning nap, substituting a nap after lunch (which also eliminates the afternoon nap). This will only work if the child is ready to give up some naptime.

If you want to be more gradual in your rearrangement of naps, cut the morning nap by ten minutes each day. Within a week or two, your child can eliminate the morning nap. Or you can start in the afternoon and cut that nap by ten minutes each day. Fairly soon the afternoon nap will be eliminated. All these modifications should be done judiciously by observing the child. If your child becomes whiny and fretful, backtrack a bit and encourage the child to sleep just after lunchtime.

The homeopathic remedy 6c/x Chamomilla is indicated when a child is especially irritable, fretful or teething. Chamomilla is especially good for children who have a hard time falling asleep and getting back to sleep when awakened.

Child Insists on Napping Late in the Day

If your child is taking a second nap in the afternoon between 4 and 6 P.M., it usually means he will have a hard time falling asleep at a normal bedtime.

The best solution is to shift naptimes around. Gradually wean your child away from a morning nap by either skipping it entirely or deducting ten minutes each day for a week or two until it is eliminated. Encourage the child to take one nap after lunchtime.

The Child Is Not Napping Enough

Some small children won't take a needed nap because they are overexcited, irritable or worried about something. Fortunately, there are two homeopathic remedies to choose from.

For a child who is probably hyperactive and who can't sleep because he is in a state of excitement or has too many ideas flowing through his head, homeopathic Coffea is indicated. Dissolve one tablet of homeopathic 3c/x or 6c/x Coffea in a tablespoon of water and give to the child in an eye dropper or in water.

If an infant won't sleep because of irritability or is very sleepy but still won't or can't fall asleep, homeopathic 6c/x Chamomilla is indicated. Give to the child in the same manner.

At-a-Glance Chart of Toddlers and Children Natural Sleep Remedies

For a complete discussion of both homeopathic remedies and tissue salts, see Chapter 7. When administering the homeopathic remedies listed in the following chart, give the child 1 tablet of 3c/x, 6c/x. 9c/x or 12c/x under the tongue and firmly instruct him to let it dissolve; make sure she doesn't chew it. For the tissue salts listed in the following chart, give 2 tablets under the tongue with the same instruction.

Note that throughout this chart the abbreviation H stands for homeopathic remedy and TS stands for tissue salts. Dosage sizes have been abbreviated to read, for example, "6c/x"; however, when buying them, you must ask for either 6c or 6x.

TODDLERS AND CHILDREN HEALTH/SLEEP PROBLEMS	NATURAL REMEDIES
GENERAL	• Water therapy: Each night give child warm, relaxing bath. This is also good strategy when child is irritable, restless or crying. Strong bedtime routine is important. • Herbal helps: Sleepless children respond to such herbal teas as catnip and chamomile. • Read Part III, Natural Remedies.
INABILITY TO SLEEP Sleeplessness. Tantrums and fussing interfere with child's ability to fall asleep.	2 tablets TS 6c/x Kali Phos.
Sleepless after excitement.	2 tablets TS 6c/x Ferrum Phos. and/or Nat. Phos.
Sleepless from nervous causes.	2 tablets TS 6c/x Kali Phos.
Awakens between midnight and 3 A.M.	1 tablet H 6c/x Arsenicum every 3 to 4 hours.
Goes to sleep easily but awakens between 3 and 4 A.M., stays awake until morning, then falls asleep.	1 tablet H 3c/x or 6c/x Nux Vomica 2 times a day for 2 weeks.
Won't go to sleep unless rocked.	Use training technique described in At-a-Glance Chart in Chapter 5.
Can't sleep because worries a lot about recent events at home or daycare/school. Filled with anxieties. Might be worried about possible nightmare.	2 tablets TS 6c/x Ferrum Phos. or Kali Phos.

Toddlers and Children Health/Sleep Problems	Natural Remedies
Can't sleep because of itching.	• Water therapy: Give child bath with several tablespoons to a cup of colloidal oatmeal (Aveeno) for sale in drugstores. If not available, place handful of organic oatmeal in the blender, reduce to powder and add to bathwater. • 2 tablets TS 6c/x Nat. Phos.
DURING-SLEEP PROBLEMS Muscles twitch before falling asleep.	2 tablets TS 6c/x Kali Phos.
Twitches during sleep.	2 tablets TS 6c/x Nat. Sulph.
Bedwetting during dreams or nightmares; feels better after nap.	1 tablet H 6c/x Equisetum at bedtime for 14 nights.
Bedwetting just after falling asleep.	1 tablet H 6c/x Causticum at bedtime for 14 nights.
Screaming during sleep with fright or wakes up screaming from a sound sleep.	2 tablets TS 6c/x Kali Phos. If asleep, don't wake up child to give remedy. Give at next bedtime.
Screams during sleep.	2 tablets TS 6c/x Nat. Phos. Don't wake up. Give at next bedtime.
Cries out during sleep.	2 tablets TS 6c/x Calcarea Phos. Don't wake up. Give at next bedtime.
Awakened from sleep by gas (flatulence).	• 2 tablets TS 6c/x Nat. Sulph. • Herbs: Make tea of bruised anise, dill or caraway seed, strain and add to water.

TODDLERS AND CHILDREN HEALTH/SLEEP PROBLEMS	NATURAL REMEDIES
Moves suddenly and involuntarily (starts) during sleep.	2 tablets TS 6c/x Nat. Mur.
Frequent dreams and exclamations during sleep.	2 tablets TS 6c/x Silica.
SLEEPWALKING Common between ages of 5 and 10; runs in families.	• Don't ask what is the matter; gently guide child back to bed. • 2 tablets TS 6c/x Kali Phos. every night. • 1 tablet H 30c/x Silica at bedtime for 2 weeks (works well if child is thin and has a large head). • If child also has night terrors and fidgety hands, give 1 tablet H 30c/x Kali Brom. at bedtime for 2 weeks. If no improvement, consult professional homeopath. • Until problem is resolved, accident-proof house: Open windows from top, not bottom. Make sure child's room is clear of obstacles. Put gate at top of stairs. Put unreachable bolt on outside door. • If appears to be related to emotional problem, consult professional therapist.
Grits teeth during sleep.	2 tablets TS 6c/x Nat. Phos.
Overresponse to noise during night and in morning.	• Insulate room from noise with drapes and/or screens, or move child to quieter room away from household and traffic noise. • Use white noise machine.

Toddlers and Children Health/Sleep Problems	Natural Remedies
	• 1 tablet H 6c/x Nux Vomica for child unusually sensitive to noise or easily irritated by any disruption. • 1 tablet H 6c/x Coffea for hyper-sensitivity to sound. • 1 tablet H 6c/x Ignatia for light sleepers who react to every disturbance.
Dribbles saliva on pillow. Possible bad breath from inflamed gums, sinus infection or tonsillitis.	1 tablet H 6c/x Merc. Sol. 3 times a day up to 7 days.
Restless sleeping and scratches anus (suspect worms).	• 2 tablets TS 6c/x Calcarea Phos. or Nat. Phos. • Herbs: Mash fresh clove of garlic, steep in honey and give several times a day up to 2 weeks. Wash out mouth after eating. (Garlic is excellent antiseptic and destroys parasites and bacteria.) • Or give garlic oil capsules. • Add acidophilus or bifidus strain of yogurt or supplements to diet to replace normal intestinal flora. • Test for pinworms: Check child's rectum with a flashlight at night. Ask your pediatrician for special tape that can be put in the child's rectum to "catch" worms so you can appraise situation.
Teething causes child to toss and turn during night. Pain may frighten child.	1 tablet H 30c/x Aconite every 30 minutes until child feels better, but not more than 10 doses.

Toddlers and Children Health/Sleep Problems	Natural Remedies
Pacifier falls out of mouth during sleep and awakens child.	• Wean child away from pacifier during daylight hours and naps. • If child is fussy during transition, give 2 tablets TS 6c/x Kali Phos.
Teething problems cause moans during sleep and irritability upon awakening.	1 tablet H 30c/x Chamomilla 1 hour before bedtime and every 30 minutes if child awakens from sleep up to 10 doses.
Demands to be in bed with parents or if child expresses fear of the dark and insists on going into parents' bed.	• 1 tablet H 6c/x Pulsatilla. • Review related Scenario above.
DREAMING Many dreams about school or quarrels.	1 tablet H 6c/x Nux Vomica.
Sleep disturbed by scary dreams.	1 tablet H 6c/x Argentum Nit.
Anxious, deep, heavy dreams.	2 tablets TS 6c/x Nat. Sulph.
Exclamations during dreams, also frequent dreams.	2 tablets TS 6c/x Silica.
Unusually strong or vivid dreams.	2 tablets TS 6c/x Calcarea Phos.
NIGHTMARES Worries and concerns that emerge during sleep and often disrupt sleep.	• Brew a tea of German Chamomile flowers (not Roman Chamomile), steep, cool, strain and have child drink. • It greatly helps child if you can talk about nightmares during the day. Ask child to tell you dream and what was scary. Encourage child to explore worries

Toddlers and Children Health/Sleep Problems	Natural Remedies
	out loud. Tell child you had scary, spooky or frightening dreams when you were a child. Reassure child about his safety and that you understand how he feels. (See scenario in text.) • Examine any recent changes in lifestyle, daycare or school, family members or neighbors that might be causing anxiety and talk about them. • Does child have separation anxiety? If you think so, give 1 tablet H 6c/x Pulsatilla every 3 to 4 hours up to 10 doses. • Play games that convey trust and safety.
Nightmares with tossing and turning and great fear.	1 tablet H 6c/x Aconite 1 hour before bedtime each night. Repeat if child wakes up and cannot go back to sleep.
Bedwetting during dreams or nightmares.	• 1 tablet H 6c/x Equisetum for 14 nights. • 2 tablets TS 6c/x alternating Ferrum Phos., Kali Phos. and Nat. Phos.
Nightmares with indigestion.	2 tablets TS 6c/x Kali Sulph. and/ or Nat. Sulph.
Nightmares about parents leaving.	• 1 tablet H 6c/x Pulsatilla. • Abandonment common fear; use related scenario in this chapter.
Shock from injury creates tendency to have bad dreams.	1 tablet H 6c/x Arnica 4 times a day up to 14 days.

TODDLERS AND CHILDREN HEALTH/SLEEP PROBLEMS	NATURAL REMEDIES
NIGHT TERRORS Frightening incidents in which child screams, sits up but is actually not awake and has no memory of incident later.	• Don't ask what's the matter; just give gentle reassurance. • 2 tablets TS 6c/x Kali Phos. (Can be given on long-term basis for sleepwalking, night terrors, awakening from sleep and screaming from fright.)
NAPS	If child has a sleep problem at night but no trouble taking a nap and going to sleep on his own, you will have less trouble changing this child's sleep pattern and getting him to fall asleep alone at night.
Too many naps during day interfere with ability to sleep at night.	• Shift and shorten naptimes. Skip early nap and have child nap right after lunch. If resists, cut morning nap by 10 minutes each day and eliminate within a week or two. Or gradually delay morning nap until afternoon. Each day cut afternoon nap by 10 minutes so you can eventually eliminate it. However, eliminating naps sometimes makes a child testy so plan a nap after lunch. Child on her own will increase nighttime sleep to compensate for shorter naptimes. • 1 tablet H 6c/x Chamomilla when child is fretful and irritable.
Can't sleep except in short nap periods and gets up feeling unrefreshed and tired.	1 tablet H 6c/x Phosphorus every 3 to 4 hours.

Toddlers and Children Health/Sleep Problems	Natural Remedies
Restless, unrefreshed sleep. Strong desire to sleep but gets up tired.	2 tablets TS 6c/x Nat. Mur.
SLEEPY OR DROWSY DURING NORMAL AWAKE TIMES Wakes up too late and is cranky when awakened (owl with late-phase sleep pattern).	Follow scenario in text. Be sure to begin new schedule during vacation time, do not allow extra nap-time and follow same schedule on weekends.
Sleepy when should be awake and lively or wakes up sleepy after a night's sleep.	• 2 tablets TS 6c/x Nat. Mur. • Can alternate with 2 tablets TS 6c/x Silica.
Hard to awaken in morning.	2 tablets TS 6c/x Calcarea Phos.
Drowsy with fever in afternoon but can't go to sleep at night.	2 tablets TS 6c/x Ferrum Phos. every 2 to 3 hours.
Drowsy in afternoon.	2 tablets TS 6c/x Ferrum Phos.
Drowsiness during day with stomach troubles or symptoms of indigestion.	2 tablets TS 6c/x Nat. Sulph. every 3 to 4 hours.
Feels and acts sleepy but cannot fall asleep.	1 tablet H 6c/x Chamomilla every 2 to 3 hours.
INAPPROPRIATE WAKEFULNESS Generally awake when it is time to sleep.	2 tablets TS 6c/x Kali Phos. and Ferrum Phos.
Resists going to sleep because of separation anxiety.	1 tablet H 6c/x Pulsatilla.

TODDLERS AND CHILDREN HEALTH/SLEEP PROBLEMS	NATURAL REMEDIES
Takes too many naps during day and can't sleep at night.	Good time to nap is right after lunchtime as it doesn't usually interfere with nighttime sleep.
Sleepy during the day but wakeful at night.	2 tablets TS 6c/x Calcarea Sulph.
Wakes up and needs to eat first thing in the morning.	Delay feeding by 10 minutes each morning. Child will soon develop another schedule, probably falling asleep again, possibly for another hour or two.
Insists on being carried around usually before bedtime.	2 tablets TS 6c/x Kali Phos.
Wide awake and irritable during first part of night and wants to be carried around.	1 tablet H 30c/x Chamomilla.
Usually awakens around 3 or 4 A.M., can't fall asleep until dawn and wakes up very tired.	1 tablet H 6c/x Nux Vomica.
Wakes up too early every morning (lark with early-phase sleep syndrome).	• Determine if actually needs less sleep. • Deliberately delay your early morning response to child by 10 minutes. • Evaluate if sleep problem is connected to too-early morning naptime. If child is old enough, gradually eliminate this nap. • Keep child's room dark in morning to help him sleep.
NOISE • Awakened by and sensitive to most noise.	• Reduce all possible stress factors: mask outside noise with

Toddlers and Children Health/Sleep Problems	Natural Remedies
	white noise machine, put child in less noisy room or add heavy curtains or barrier near bed to stop outside or household noise.
• Light sleeper who reacts to every disturbance.	• 1 tablet H 6c/x Ignatia.
• Oversensitive to sounds.	• 1 tablet H 6c/x Coffea.
• Oversensitive to disruption and noise.	• 1 tablet H 6c/x Nux Vomica or TS 6c/x Kali Phos.

LIGHT
Very sensitive and responsive to light in morning.

• Reduce light coming into room in morning with heavy drapes or light-reducing shades.
• 2 tablets TS 6c/x Kali Phos.

MEDICAL AND OTHER SITUA-TIONS AFFECTING SLEEP
BEDWETTING
Most 2- and 3-year-olds wet their bed occasionally. After 6, consistent bedwetting should be investigated. About 75% of consistent bedwetters over 7 (most are boys) may have inherited a bedwetting gene, says Dr. Hans Elberg of the University of Copenhagen. Sometimes bedwetting occurs after a child has been dry for a while because of a special circumstance like a shock, scare, period of coughing or newly developed food sensitivity (test by eliminating milk products and, if that doesn't work, wheat products).

• Water therapy: Whether child has primary or secondary incontinence, German hydrotherapy will toughen and strengthen healthy child. Make a game of dipping younger child in and out of cold water for a second or two, then immediately envelop child in large, cozy towel. For children over 4 or 5, run cold water in tub high enough to cover child's calves and have child walk in the water while you hold on. Start with only a few seconds and work up to 5 minutes a day.
• Herbal teas: To allay anxiety, make up combination of linden, chamomile and catnip tea to drink in late afternoon before dinner.

Toddlers and Children Health/Sleep Problems	Natural Remedies
	• Behavior modification: You can buy sensor for sheet which rings bell and awakens child whenever moisture is discovered (see Resources). • Restrict beverages after middle of afternoon, and make sure child urinates just before going to bed. • Be quick to take this child to the bathroom if he awakens during night and first thing in the morning. • If you suspect a urinary infection, check with pediatrician.
Wets bed just after falling asleep.	• Child's dose H 6c/x Causticum at bedtime up to 14 nights. • Alternate 2 tablets TS 6c/x Ferrum Phos., Kali Phos. or Nat. Phos. every 3 hours for a few weeks.
Wets bed during dreams or nightmares.	• 1 tablet H 6c/x Equisetum at bedtime. Can repeat dose up to 14 nights. • 2 tablets TS 6c/x Ferrum Phos., Kali Phos. or Nat. Phos. every 3 hours for several weeks.
CONSTIPATION	• Water therapy: Cold water starts persistalsis. Give child cool water to drink first thing every morning to avoid constipation. • When severely constipated, pediatricians suggest use of suppositories and retraining child to pass stool at least once every other day and then every day.

- Add fiber to diet to keep stool soft.
- Other stool softeners are 5 to 10 drops of organic flaxseed, black current seed or borage oil added to foods. Or add liquid food-grade aloe juice drops to apple juice or apple sauce several times a day.

CRYING FITS

- 2 tablets TS 6c/x Kali Phos.
- Herbal teas: Add tablespoon of either linden (limeflowers) or chamomile flower tea to water. Other calming teas are caraway seed, catnip, fennel seed and ginger.
- Experiment with Bach flower remedies: Chicory, Walnut or Rescue Remedy. Put drops diluted in tablespoon of water on forehead and/or under tongue.
- Pressure point: Whenever child is restless or crying, gently scratch backs of her hands.
- Massage hands and feet.

DIARRHEA
Loose bowels affects child's ability to sleep.

- Adequate fluid intake is essential to prevent dehydration. Start with clear liquids such as water or ice chips, cooled ginger tea or tiny sips of flat Classic Coke or 7-Up, Gatorade or pure Coca Cola syrup (available by mail from Heritage; see Resources).
- For nausea/diarrhea, coat the stomach with gelatin dessert and slowly add dry crackers or cereal.

TODDLERS AND CHILDREN HEALTH/SLEEP PROBLEMS	NATURAL REMEDIES
	• When diarrhea stops, try TRABY diet: toast, rice, applesauce, bananas and yogurt. (Avoid milk, but active acidophilus yogurt is usually well accepted.) • Massage hands and feet.
DIGESTIVE PROBLEMS Drowsy and sleepy during day with abdominal discomfort, nausea, headache or constipation. Tongue has green-gray or brown-green coating.	2 tablets TS 6c/x Nat. Sulph. every 3 to 4 hours.
Very sleepy and drowsy during day because of digestive problems which affect ability to sleep.	2 tablets TS 6c/x Nat. Sulph. every 3 to 4 hours.
Nightmares because of indigestion.	2 tablets TS 6c/x Kali Sulph. or Nat. Sulph.
Overeating during day affects ability to sleep.	1 tablet H 6c/x Pulsatilla every 3 to 4 hours.
Rubs eyes and acts as if throat is parched or you suspect some dehydration because of illness or vomiting.	• 2 tablets TS 6c/x Nat. Mur. • Give child additional water to drink during day.
EMOTIONAL PROBLEMS Daytime fears show up at night.	• Some children act out daytime fears such as deep-rooted separation anxieties and fear of abandonment just as they are going to sleep. They need great deal of daily reassurance.

Toddlers and Children Health/Sleep Problems	Natural Remedies
	• For children who fear abandonment or separation from parents, 1 tablet H 6c/x Pulsatilla every 3 to 4 hours up to 10 doses, as needed.
Problem with sibling or friends at day care.	1 tablet H 6c/x Nux Vomica every 2 to 3 hours up to 10 doses, as needed.
Grief after some beloved person dies.	If child is in a terrible state of grief, 1 tablet H 6c/x Ignatia every 3 to 4 hours up to 10 doses as needed.
Overexcitement can prevent child from falling asleep.	• 2 tablets TS 6c/x Ferrum Phos. and/or Nat. Phos. • Chamomile flower tea tranquilizes. If child is unduly excited, add 1 to 2 drops of valerian tincture to tea.
FEVER Nature's weapon against infection. High or low fever.	• Water therapy is safest, quickest, most natural antidote to fever. Give child cool water to drink; the more cool water, the quicker the fever is reduced. • Cold friction rub with washcloth dipped into cold water, apple cider vinegar or chamomile tea (see description in Chapter 9). Increases inner circulation and starts internal healing process. • A tea of 1 teaspoon raspberry jam is useful fever antidote.
Feverish child sleeps in afternoon but cannot sleep at night.	2 tablets TS 6c/x Ferrum Phos. every 3 to 4 hours.

TODDLERS AND CHILDREN HEALTH/SLEEP PROBLEMS	NATURAL REMEDIES
FUSSY Grumpy, cross and can't go to sleep.	• 2 tablets TS 6c/x Kali Phos. • Drink glass of water with one teaspoon of honey and apple cider vinegar. Can be sipped during day. • Most children relax in leisurely warm bath.
ILL-TEMPERED Before and while going to sleep.	2 tablets TS 6c/x Kali Phos.
LOW SPIRITS Acts as if everything is hopeless.	2 tablets TS 6c/x Nat. Mur.
NERVOUS Periods of great nervous tension with interludes of yawning.	2 tablets TS 6c/x Magnesia Phos. every 3 to 4 hours.
Insomnia from physical or mental exhaustion or excitement.	2 tablets TS 6c/x Kali Phos. every 3 to 4 hours.
Some children review events of day and worry about them. Others worry about events of next day, especially class event, play or oral report (sleepless version of stage fright).	• 1 tablet H 6c/x Lycopodium before bedtime every 2 hours up to 10 doses. • Bach flower remedy: White Chestnut. Add 4 drops to teaspoon of cool water and place under tongue when worry gets obsessively repetitive.
OVEREXCITED Too excited to sleep.	1 tablet TS 6c/x Ferrum Phos. and/or Nat. Phos.
OVERTENSE Mind is overactive from exhaustion and stress so toss and turn and can't sleep.	1 tablet H 6c/x Coffea 1 hour before bedtime. Can be repeated every 3 to 4 hours as needed.

Toddlers and Children Health/Sleep Problems	Natural Remedies
SHOCK Can't sleep because of fright or shock. If child falls asleep, may have nightmares.	1 tablet H 6c/x Aconite every 3 to 4 hours up to 10 doses, as needed.
Emotional shock causes continual yawning.	1 tablet H 6c/x Ignatia 1 hour before bedtime for 10 days.
Grief from loss of beloved relative, friend or neighbor causes insomnia.	1 tablet H 6c/x Ignatia every 3 to 4 hours up to 10 doses, as needed.
Loss of close person causes restless sleep.	1 tablet H 6c/x Aconite up to 10 doses.
Bruising pain from injury leads to bad dreams.	1 tablet H 6c/x Arnica 4 times a day up to 14 days.
TOOTHACHE Severe shooting pain makes it difficult to sleep.	1 tablet H 6c/x Coffea every 5 minutes up to 10 doses.

7

Teens Require More Sleep.

From birth onward the pineal gland releases the hormone melatonin, which controls the rhythm of our waking and sleeping. Since babies produce prodigious quantities of melatonin, they sleep most of the day and night. Gradually the production of melatonin peaks by age six as the need for long periods of sleep lessens and more waking hours are needed, and after that, one's body begins secreting less melatonin. This changes again at puberty, sometime between ages 11 and 14, and continues for the next six to ten years. When puberty starts, the gradual decrease of melatonin stops, and there is a sudden, precipitous downward jolt in production. Scientists conjecture that this abrupt plunge may be the reason teenagers have a biological inclination to go to sleep later than when they were preteens. Teens, even larks who always got up early in the morning, now have a tendency to get up later. This change in scheduling—later to bed, later to rise—doesn't mean teenagers need less sleep; studies show that teens actually crave more sleep than before. Adequate sleep is vital for teens for a wide variety of reasons, but especially the release of growth hormones which occurs most often during sleep. The impact of sleep deprivation on good moods and good grades is self-evident.

Dr. Mary Carskadon, a chronobiologist at Brown University School of Medicine in Providence, Rhode Island, who has spent the last twenty-five years investigating the vagaries of adolescent sleep, concludes that teenagers are biologically programmed to sleep about 9 1/2 hours a night. Contrast this with the amount most teenagers actually get each night—6 hours on the average—and no wonder most kids are sleep-starved. These biological imperatives put the teenager in ironic conflict with the world in which he lives. Biology demands that the teenager get to sleep later and get up later than before. However, American junior and senior highs all start as early as 7 A.M., one and a half to two hours earlier than elementary schools! This demand for alertness early in the morning comes at a time when the teenager's biology programs her to be fast asleep.

Puberty from age 11 or later is a time of enormous growth and mental development, with rapid changes in body size and shape. This is a time of life that demands clear, persistent thinking and memory. It is also a period of intellectual and physical ferment. New hobbies are born. Sports activities take time and physical effort. Music of all kinds becomes important. Homework is demanding and time consuming. Home chores need to be done. Some teens work at outside jobs—as baby sitters or in nighttime retail establishments. At the very time the entire group needs more sleep, school, home and outside demands prevent sleep and are responsible for less sleeptime. An American teenager who has to be in school at 7 A.M., often has to get up about 5:30 A.M. According to a report from the Center for Narcolepsy Research, College of Nursing, University of Illinois at Chicago, "Over a period of several nights of getting 5 to 6 hours of sleep, a 'sleep debt' of 2 or 3 hours per night begins to build up." Researchers on teenage sleep say that a sleep debt leads to:

- Less daytime alertness.
- Difficulties with memory and reasoning tasks.
- Slower reaction times in braking a car.
- Possible mood swings and abrupt irritation.

Dr. Carskadon and her colleague Dr. Amy Wolfson of the College of Holy Cross in Worcester, Massachusetts, as well as other prominent American sleep scientists, are urging school systems throughout the United States to rethink school and bus schedules. Dr. Carskadon and others have been holding task force meetings on the impact on teenage learning of early school openings. The first series of meetings suggested an exchange of elementary school opening times with junior and senior high openings. This could give sleep-deprived adolescents a later, more "natural" arrival in keeping with their inherent biological needs. Dr. Carskadon also urges teens to take responsibility for their own sleep habits and to try to squeeze in more daily sleep. Dr. Carskadon claims if teens manage to get enough sleep for only one week they will notice both a marked difference in memory, mood, concentration and good humor and the fact that sleep helps them overcome hostility and defensiveness.

Professor Peretz Lavie, Dean of the Rappaport Faculty of Medicine, who headed a study conducted by the Technion-Israel Institute of Technology, presented a paper at the 9th Annual Meeting of the American Sleep Disorders Association and the Sleep Research Society held in Nashville, Tennessee, in 1995. His group analyzed data on student sleeping patterns in 13 countries in the developed world. The results showed that Israeli students started school earlier (7:30 A.M.) than many of their peers in other countries. In extensive studies of student behavior and teacher reports, the researchers found that when students start a school day too early, they have difficulty concentrating and are irritable. "The negative effects of an early-starting school day carry over into family life, creating tension and stress between parents and irritable children," says Professor Lavie. Because of the study, the Israeli Ministry of Education delayed the official start of classes until 8 A.M. Followup research showed that starting the school day later made children less disruptive and more able to focus better.

Getting Teens to Make a Sleep Contract

Dr. Ronald E. Dahl at the University of Pittsburgh School of Medicine has written extensively on child and adolescent sleep problems. He works successfully with teenagers with mild to extreme disorders. "The most common cause of mild-to-moderate sleepiness in adolescents is an inadequate number of hours in bed," says Dr. Dahl. "A combination of social schedules leading to late nights with early-morning school requirements can significantly compress the number of hours of sleep. Part-time jobs, sports activities, hobbies and active social lives can exacerbate this problem. Catch-up sleep on weekends and holidays and a diet of naps can further contribute to the problem by leading to erratic schedules and even later nights."

Dr. Dahl points out that significant gains are made by involving the entire family in identifying and understanding the problem of adolescent sleep deprivation and in helping students go to sleep earlier. He has the students as well as the parents analyze these basic questions:

- How sleep-deprived is the student?
- Is there disturbed sleep during the night?
- If the student is actually getting enough sleep, does he or she have special requirement for additional sleep?
- Is there a biorhythm clock problem?
- Is there a scheduling problem?
- Are there any sleep disorders (such as sleep apnea or narcolepsy)?

Dr. Dahl helps the student and family analyze all the causes of the sleep problems. When the student agrees that he needs to change his lifestyle in order to acquire more sleep, the next step is a behavioral contract that is then signed by the teenager.

In order to work out a unique contract for each teenager, Dr. Dahl and the teenager amass a list of specific problems that may possibly cause bad sleep habits. These may include some or all of the following late-afternoon or evening activities that influence sleeptime: a job, during-the-week sports, club or social activities, homework, hobbies, video game playing, phone calls, listening to music, television watching, Internet browsing, eating heavy meals late at night, erratic (times or places) napping, oversleeping in the morning that makes students late for school, problems getting to school, use of alcohol, caffeine products or sleeping pills, and so on. On the basis of the list that emerges, Dr. Dahl suggests and negotiates changes in the daily schedule based on a variety of choices that can be made. The final contract lists the following decisions:

- The exact time the teenager agrees to go to bed each night. (Dr. Dahl allows only small deviations on the weekend.)
- Rewards for successes (which the teenager is interested in attaining).
- Negative consequences for failures.

Dealing with Mild to Moderate Problems

Dr. Dahl and the teenager work out a new schedule with consistent, gradual 15-minute-a-day changes in bedtime and waketime. The optimal sleeptime picked is one when the adolescent can go to sleep without difficulty. Then that time is decreased each day by 15 minutes until a desirable time for sleep is arrived at—say, 10 or 11 P.M. Two things are important to keep in mind during this period of change and adjustment of sleep habits: avoid naps and be consistent with sleep and waketimes on weekends and holidays.

More Severe Sleep Problems: Phase-Delayed Sleep Syndrome

Certain teenagers complain that they cannot fall asleep until 3 or 5 A.M. and then they have a lot of trouble getting out of bed for school. Youngsters and others who develop this erratic clock problem (a phase-delayed sleep syndrome) often take a late afternoon nap, which then prevents them from getting to bed early. Dr. Dahl's treatment for this syndrome consists of two parts: gradually getting the body's sleep system on a new, more desirable schedule and maintaining that new schedule.

Severe Cases of Resistant Sleeplessness

"In some severe cases, adolescents on very late schedules respond more favorably to going around the clock without sleep with successive delays in bedtime," says Dr. Dahl. For these cases he suggests the following schedule: moving sleeptime ahead by three hours each day for a week:

Day One: Stay up until 6 A.M. and sleep until 3:00 P.M.
Day Two: Go to bed at 9 A.M. and sleep until 6 P.M.
Day Three: Go to bed at noon and sleep until 9 P.M.
Day Four: Go to bed at 3 P.M. and sleep until midnight.
Day Five: Go to bed at 6 P.M. and sleep until 3 A.M.
Day Six: Go to bed at 9 P.M. and sleep until 6 A.M.
Day Seven: Go to sleep at 10 P.M. and sleep until 7 A.M.

At the end of the week the teenagers should be on a comfortable sleep schedule that conforms to school schedules and other needs.

Solving Special Teen Sleep Problems

Teens can also be subject to other sleep problems, especially scary nightmares or night terrors. A number of natural remedies can help alleviate them.

NIGHTMARES

Nightmares that persist from childhood can terrorize a teen and prevent sleep. Common nightmares include enemies that change in shape, character, size and place or frightening dreams that are repeated over and over. Read the section on reworking nightmares with different, more acceptable endings described under Mental Exercises in Chapter 10. Review the tissue salts and homeopathic remedies that offset nightmares in the chart in Chapter 5 as well as the general discussion of such nature-based remedies in Chapter 8.

NIGHT TERRORS

Night terrors, in which children scream and shriek with fright but are not actually awake, usually disappear by age twelve. However, they can erupt again in adolescence as well as in adulthood when a person is under great stress or after the use of alcohol or drugs.

To solve the problem, convene a family pow-wow to analyze the stresses in the youngster's life. Decide together how the stresses can be met and eased. Work out a comfortable, consistent day and evening schedule with acceptable yet firm going-to-sleep hours. If the night terrors persist, make sure the youngster goes to sleep earlier than before and awaken him during the first hour of sleep (terrors only occur during that time. To overcome continuing mental strain, use any of the relaxing herbal teas and take two to five pellets (number depends on the size and weight of the teen) 6c/x tissue salt Kali Phos. (See Chapter 8 for a thorough discussion of tissue salts and other nature-based medicines.)

General Sleep Tips for Teens

- Determine your minimum requirements for sleep. The average need for most teenagers is 8 to 8½ hours every night. However, some teenagers function well on 6 or 7. Others need 9½ hours. Strive to achieve your minimum requirements.
- Instead of doing homework late at night, wake up earlier in the morning and do it then.
- Avoid stimulants such as colas, coffee, tea and cigarettes (see Chapter 2).
- People function better and sleep better when they include a mild exercise program in their daily life. If you're not getting exercise as part of school, then fit some exercise—fast walking, swimming, rollerblading—into your daily routine. Remember it's better to exercise in the morning; late night exercise is too stimulating.
- Don't drink liquor; alcohol creates rebound insomnia (see Chapter 2).
- Never take sleeping pills: they only work for a short while and then create additional sleeping problems (see Chapter 2).
- To calm down before sleep, drink a half cup of such herbal teas as chamomile, hops, passionflower and valerian (see Chapter 8).
- Take a warm bath in the evening to promote sleep.
- Practice yawning or try any of the other physical or mental exercises discussed in Chapter 10.
- Use of homeopathic remedies and tissue salts depends on the teenager's height, size and weight. For small-bodied, younger teens follow the recommendations in Chapter 6. Taller, older teenagers may find it more useful to follow the suggestions in Chapter 4.

PART

III

Natural Sleep Remedies

In some ways 1972 was a crucial year for natural medicine. It was the year President Richard Nixon made his breakthrough visit to China, and *The New York Times* correspondent who accompanied him had an appendicitis attack. That wouldn't normally be news, but the journalist wrote about his experience with Chinese pain relief. Suddenly, a large part of the Western world became informed about the 4,000-year-old Chinese system of medicine called "acupuncture." In acupuncture, hair-thin needles are inserted at one or many of 500 skin points in order to stimulate and release the master energy force called "chi" that heals and balances the body. The Chinese also use hundreds of common plants for healing. These ancient Chinese systems defied analysis by our modern approach to medicine, at least in 1972. Among the eminent physicians who eventually went to China to study acupuncture was the world-famous ear surgeon, Dr. Samuel Rosen, who wrote these prophetic words: "I have seen the past—and it works."

Since the 1930s Western medicine systematically discarded the use of plants for healing and scoffed at every traditional approach to health and healing. So *The New York Times* story in 1972 broke a cultural log-jam. Since then, thousands of books and articles have been published on the many different kinds of natural medicine. Millions of people have rediscovered the usable past and found there were countless safe, alternative, complementary and nondrug approaches that could release blocked energy, cure and prevent illnesses and promote good health. Without dislodging their connections to Western-trained allopathic doctors, millions of people in Europe and the United States quietly sought preventive health measures from research-oriented nutritionists, chiropractors, naturopaths, homeopaths and body workers in a variety of disciplines. In this guide to natural sleep we bring all the pertinent, safe, self-care, nondrug modalities together in one place for the first time.

8

Nature-Based Medicines

Since prehistoric times, plants have been used as nature's primary medicine chest. By trial and error, ancient peoples on every continent used leaves, stems, bark, flowers, fruits, seeds and roots to get the body to respond in a healthy biologic fashion. Half of today's medicines are chemical duplications of ancient plant remedies. For instance, reserpine, one of the world's first tranquilizer drugs, is the chemical clone of the African root rauwolfia, first used by African tribal healers. When early North American explorers contracted deadly scurvy, Native Americans saved their lives with vitamin C-rich brews of spruce tree needles. These same Native Americans astonished early visitors with their sophisticated use of blackberry thorns and brambles to superficially inject medicines into the skin. Explorers and pioneers also learned from Native Americans how to use the inner bark of the willow tree to reduce respiratory infections and inflammations. Much later the chemical code for willow bark was broken when a German chemist created aspirin.

In this chapter we will discuss four different ways that natural substances have been found to heal the body and promote relaxing, restorative sleep, including herbal medicine, homeopathy, tissue or cell salts and Bach flower remedies.

Herbal Medicine

Ethnobotanist James Duke, once Chief of the Medicinal Plant Resources Laboratory, U.S. Department of Agriculture (USDA), says, "There are about 12,000 licensed homeopaths and naturopaths who routinely use herbal remedies in the United States. In other parts of the world, as much as 90 percent of the population relies on traditional medicines, mostly herbal." Most herbs are available as fresh and dried plants, in tinctures and essential oils, frequently as pills and sometimes as "waters" (orange buds and lavender). Used both internally and externally, most herbs can either be brewed as infusions or decoctions or used as foot or whole baths or in combinations as poultices or compresses. Three aromatic herbs—flowers of hops, lavender and mignonette—may be encased in pillows to induce sleep. The herbs chamomile, passionflower and valerian are also available as homeopathic remedies. Various national and international producers also sell teething and colic remedies of homeopathic chamomile.

While some people may prefer to consult an experienced herbal practitioner, it is possible to learn about herbs and how to use them safely and successfully on your own. If you tend to be allergic, or haven't used one of the herbs discussed here before, experiment with a small dose to note your reaction. Once you find you can use an herb, you can combine two or more herbs as needed. However, it may help to keep in mind that herbs are slow acting and certain precautions, as noted below, may apply.

THE MANY WAYS YOU CAN USE HERBS

Soothing and relaxing herbs can be taken internally or applied externally in the following ways:

- To make an *infusion* (tea), add flowers, leaves or aerial parts of the herb to boiling water. Unless otherwise noted, use a handful of the fresh herb or a tablespoon of the dried herb to a cup of boiling water. Steep from five to ten minutes or longer. Strain out the herb. If you make larger amounts, store it in the refrigerator in a labeled glass jar as infusions are perishable.
- Roots, barks and seeds normally must be simmered for twenty minutes to a half hour to make a *decoction*. (When you make a chicken soup you're making a decoction.) Use a handful of the herb to four cups of water. Steep for twenty minutes and strain out the herb. Store any leftover liquid in a labeled glass jar in the refrigerator.
- *Tinctures* are made by steeping flowers, leaves, aerial parts, roots, barks or seeds in an 80-proof alcohol such as vodka or gin. Use about a handful of herbs to about a pint of the liquor. I usually add the liquor to a slightly larger labeled glass jar. Place it in a dark closet to steep for a week to twenty-one days. Use after straining out plant parts twice.
- *Juleps* are made from buds or seeds such as caraway and fennel. To release the volatile oils of seeds or buds, gently press them between

your fingers before placing them in either water or milk. Use a pinch of seeds to a cup of liquid or two tablespoons to a pint. Steep between five to ten minutes or longer and strain. A handful of bruised seeds may also be steeped in a pint of vodka or gin to make a tincture (strain out after storing in a dark closet for one to three weeks).

- *Essential oils* are the concentrated essence of a plant. Sometimes the plant oils, which are extracted by distillation, are used because of their aroma; other times they are used for their medicinal or culinary value. Since essential oils are more potent than the fresh or dried plant, it is only necessary to use the oil in minuscule amounts, a few drops at a time. Many essential oils are so potent that they can irritate the skin, so they need to be placed in a carrier oil such as almond, sunflower or coconut for massage or first aid.

- Compresses, made with teas of chamomile, lavender, lemon balm (melissa) or tincture of valerian, can be applied externally to the head. Appropriate compresses help control headaches and reduce nervousness, which in turn allow for easier sleep. To make a compress, dip a folded cloth, such as a clean dish towel, into a tea, wring out and apply directly to the body to relax tight muscles or stop cramps.

- A *poultice* is similar to a compress, but the whole herb is applied instead of a liquid infusion or extract. Poultices can be applied hot or cold. To make one, chop fresh herbs in a food processor or mash herbs with some hot boiling water for a few minutes. Then place the herb directly on the skin in the desired area and secure it in place with some thin clean cotton cloth or gauze.

TYPES OF HERBS

Catnip, chamomile, hops, passionflower, scullcap and valerian are all relaxing herbs that also reduce anxiety and calm the body. Lavender, linden (American) or limeflowers (Europe), melissa (lemon balm), orange buds or orange flower and rosemary are aromatic herbs that are also relaxing and helpful for digestion as well as sleep. Each aromatic may be used singly or combined, when needed, with other, stronger sleep-promoting herbs. The aromatics may be used on a daily basis at lunch, dinner or before sleep. The culinary herb sage also has some mellowing-out abilities and a pinch may be added on occasion to other teas according to taste. Several bruised cloves and/or bruised cumin seeds may be added to any herbal tea to allay nervousness prior to sleep.

Catnip (Nepeta cataria)
Catnip is a pleasant-tasting, sedative, antispasmodic herb that was once

Herbs for Children

A variety of herbal teas can be either ingested by the nursing mother and/ or given in teaspoon doses mixed in water to the child to overcome such common sleep-disturbing problems as nightmares, colic, teething and bedwetting.

Nightmares

Chamomile, primrose, rosemary, thyme. Bruised fresh thyme may be eaten on bread as in the Arab countries to prevent nightmares or, like the other herbs, made into a tea. Homeopathic chamomile can be purchased in infant and child doses in most health food stores or through mail order sources (see Resources).

Colic

Make a julep or a tea of bruised seeds of caraway, dill or fennel or teas of angelica, catnip or chamomile. Also, use children's homeopathic pilules or pellets of chamomile.

Teething

Chamomile tea or dissolved homeopathic Chamomilla, licorice root or orris root.

Bedwetting

Make dried marjoram into a tea to be drunk in the early part of the day, or have the child eat fresh, bruised marjoram on any nonwhite bread. Since bedwetting can sometimes occur because of food sensitivities, experiment by eliminating milk as a possible culprit (replace cow's milk with soy milk), and watch for a possible sensitivity to wheat and corn products. Health food stores have many varieties of gluten-free breads to choose from.

---

used in every European and American farmhouse as a sleep tea, especially for fretful and/or flatulent babies. Little sacks of catnip were also tied around infants' necks to settle stomach problems and to help prevent nightmares. A tea of this plant is also used to calm adults before sleep, to stop hiccups and to alleviate menstrual pain. Such a tea is useful when the absence of menstrual flow or irregular flow interferes with sleep. According to ethnobotanist James Duke, "a tablespoon of the leaf juice, two or three times a day, is claimed to restore the menstrual flow when all else fails."

TEA: Don't boil catnip because it looses its volatile properties. Instead, steep a handful of the leaf sprays and flowers in a pint of boiling water and cover tightly. Take three tablespoons morning and evening. For children place a teaspoon in a water bottle to help expel wind. If the child is over a year, catnip tea can be sweetened with honey. (Never give honey to a child under one year.)

Appalachian herbalist Tommie Bass says in *Herbal Medicine Past and Present,* "It is one of the oldest there's been for babies. A tea for the baby is one of the most wonderful things. It'll pacify them and help them sleep. It will do away with the hives and if the stomach don't digest its food, why it will just start that to digesting. And it will do the same thing for grown people too, but we've got to take more of it. Yes, sir, it's a real good one." Pharmacognosy (the science of medicines from natural sources) expert Varro Tyler says also in *Herbal Medicine Past and Present,* "There just may be some basis in fact for the cup of hot catnip tea taken at bedtime to ensure a good night's sleep. Besides, it's relatively inexpensive, it tastes good, and no harmful effects from using it have been reported. What more can one ask of a beverage?"

Catnip is often combined with scullcap (*Scutellaria galerculata*), a powerful nervine plant, or placed in a combination with hops and scullcap. The British herbalist Mrs. M. Grieve reports in her 1931 classic, *A Modern Herbal,* that this last combination plus lime blossoms produces a "natural sleep" for morphine addicts.

Chamomile (German or Hungarian Matricaria recutia*)*

Chamomile flower tea is an old standby to calm and relax the body and, along with peppermint tea and lemon balm (melissa), is a frequent table tea especially in France and Spain. The Greeks loved the apple-smelling aroma of this ground-cover herb and named it "earth apple," while the Spanish called it *manzanilla,* "little apple." Over the centuries Italians have used chamomile tea to calm people before going to bed, and old country wisdom recommends that it be used one hour before bedtime by elderly people. Over the course of many hundreds of years Europeans have used chamomile as a primary aid for children's sleep problems such as nightmares (as both a preventive and a remedy) and to allay the pain of teething.

The flowers contain the most important tonic and soothing medicinal values of this versatile herb. Among its many attributes, chamomile is thought to relieve nervousness and nervous excitement in all parts of the body, including those caused by digestive problems.

TEA: Place thirty flowers of chamomile in a jug, pour a pint of boiling water over the flowers, steep for ten or fifteen minutes and strain out the flowers. Drink an hour before going to sleep. Sweeten with honey if the child is over one year of age. Add a cup of strained chamomile tea to a baby's bathwater to ensure calm and induce sleep. Chamomile is a ground cover, so to avoid the possibility of adulteration with ragweed, make sure to use only your own flowers or dried flowers from a reliable source.

TINCTURE: Early in the day use eight to sixteen drops of chamomile tincture in a cup of cold water. Sip some every hour to relieve adult neuralgic pains that emerge at night or to alleviate mild sleep problems. It is important to note that chamomile has a strong effect on babies. Add several drops of chamomile tincture to a cup of cold water, then add to a water bottle or cup to decrease and control restlessness and irritability in children and to allay the pain of teething.

ESSENTIAL OIL: Add two to three drops of the oil to bathwater for sedative and antispasmodic action.

HOMEOPATHIC CHAMOMILE: This is available as a children's remedy and is highly recommended for teething and colic.

ALERT: The essential oil of chamomile is a uterine stimulant, so be sure not to use it during pregnancy. Because of the possibility of contamination with ragweed, do not use chamomile if you have a known allergy to ragweed. Some people have contact dermatitis to the fresh plant.

Hops (Humulus lupulus)

Hops have been used since the 11th century to brew tonic ales and have been known for centuries to produce sleep when all else fails. Hops grow as a vine, and the female fruits, called "strobiles," which are cone-shaped with overlapping leaves, look like thin, elongated artichokes. Although the whole plant is considered a nervine (herbal aid to nerves) and a tonic, it is the yellow powder from the fruit that contains the most valuable medicinal assets. The young tender shoots are quite tasty and are often given to nursing mothers to increase their breast milk. This also calms down testy babies and helps them sleep. When you can obtain young, fresh hops, eat six to eight raw flowers in the morning and evening.

European varieties of hops are said to have a more sedative effect and better flavor than the American variety. As American pioneers explored the vast countryside they ate young hops as a food tonic, made hops into homemade beer and sewed fresh hops into pillows to promote restful sleep. In the last century British farm and working people made a tonic homebrew and sleep-inducing hops ale, which they drank with a very light supper of salad greens and bread and butter.

TEA: Make the hop flowers into a tea by steeping a tablespoon in a pint of cold water and simmering for ten minutes. Steep and strain out the herb. Drink two cups in the morning and early afternoon. Use the same method with freeze-dried and freshly dried hops. Old-time herbalists often added chamomile and valerian to hops tea as a sleeping potion.

TINCTURE: You can make your own sleep-inducing hops tincture. Add ten drops to boiling water to ease anxiety and tension. Or add several drops to catnip, chamomile, lemon balm, passionflower, peppermint or other relaxing table teas.

DIGESTIVE CORDIAL: Hops contains an invaluable bitter principle which works miracles for many digestive and sleep problems. To make an instant digestive cordial, steep eight to sixteen drops of hops tincture in a cup of sherry. In pioneer days people created a home hops, called "bitters," by combining 1/2 ounce of hops, 1 ounce angelica leaves or roots and 1 ounce of holy thistle and pouring one and a half quarts of boiling water on the mixture. Steep until cool, strain out the herbs, discard, reserve the liquid and label the jar: "Hops Bitters." Since angelica has a high sugar content, do not use if pregnant or diabetic.

CAPSULES: Take only for one day, then discontinue for several days.

PILLOW: The powerful aromatic effect of the hops plant is known to promote sleep. In fact, there are anecdotes about people entering hops warehouses and falling into profound sleep. It is said that George III slept on a hops pillow to distract him from the incapacitating disease porphyria.

When making a hops pillow, encase several handfuls of hops flowers in a muslin envelope. To prevent crackling sounds when you use the pillow, sprinkle the flowers with a few drops of alcohol or sleep-inducing aromatic lavender tincture. Sew the envelope closed and cover with a pillow case. Hops pillows can be "recharged" by occasionally placing them in the sun.

ALERT: Avoid ingesting this plant if you have a tendency for depression. Some people may have a contact sensitivity (they develop dermatitis) to the live plant.

Lavender (Lavandula augustifolia)

Lavender is one of the world's favorite aromatic herbs, and it is fragrant in both its fresh and dried forms. It can be purchased as dried flowers, a tincture or an aromatic essential oil. I am particularly fond of the essential oil and use drops of it on pillow cases to provide a heavenly sleep-producing scent. I also combine the oil with hops flowers when creating a hops pillow. The essential oil can be diluted with any favorite oil (I like almond) to create a marvelous body massage oil. It is useful as a natural component in sleep-inducing techniques because the aroma of the oil, when massaged into the neck and shoulders, reduces the tension of headaches and neck aches.

Fresh or dried lavender flowers can also help alleviate children's sleep problems. Create a weak infusion by steeping a tablespoon of the flowers in a cup of boiling water for five minutes, then strain out and discard the flowers. Give a child a teaspoon in an eyedropper for irritability and colic.

ALERT: Do not use lavender internally during pregnancy because it is a uterine stimulant.

Linden or limeflowers (Tilia Europaea)

Linden or limeflowers is a delicious tasting tea, called *tilleul* in France and beloved because of its aroma, flavor and sedative effect. The young flowers are often used in weak tea as an infant's drink to calm nervous babies. Teas made of the flowers also help with indigestion and extreme nervousness, even nervous vomiting. Old French country remedies include using a pint of strong tea in a warm to hot bath to overcome hysteria or nervous irritability. The tea can also be used in an enema. Bees love limeflowers, and the Europeans, especially the French, make a wonderful tilleul honey. Add it to catnip, hops, lavender, scullcap and valerian teas to enhance their sleep-inducing impact.

ALERT: When using dried flowers, check to see if they are old. If so, do not use, as old limeflowers can be a narcotic. Do not drink linden tea frequently if you have any heart problems.

Melissa/Lemon balm (Melissa officinalis)

Bees are very attracted to melissa. In fact, the very name "melissa" is Greek for "honey bee." The leaves contain the plant's medicinal principles which are cooling, refreshing, restorative for the nervous system and an antidote to worry, especially when worry or anxiety causes digestive disturbances. I always have on hand an old German compound "Melissana," which is made from an ancient recipe of Carmelite nuns. A few drops are an excellent, instant digestive, the liquid can be used externally as a body rub or a few drops can be added to a bath to relax tense muscles.

TEA: Make a tea with a handful of the fresh leaves.

TINCTURE: If you grow lemon balm, make your own tinctures with several handfuls of the washed, fresh leaves. Use five to sixteen drops of the tincture in a cup of boiling water for a relaxing, calming tea.

Passionflower (Passiflora incarnata)

Passionflower is often used in Europe and in many island cultures as a mild, hypnotic, sedative herb to calm the nervous system and promote sleep. It should not be used by someone who feels depressed, as it will intensify the depression. In the past it was actively used in America, usually in combination with other sleep herbs such as scullcap. Appalachian herbalist Tommie Bass considers it "the most wonderful sleep and pacifying plant, valuable for a nerve medicine." According to Bass in *Herbal Medicine Past and Present,* "Any good sleeping medicine has passionflower in it." Mountain people use four or five cups a day as a nerve tonic or sleep aid. "It'll cause you to sleep like a baby most every time," says Bass. He likes to combine passionflower with scullcap, peach leaves and sage and occasionally adds catnip to his sleep potion. *A Guide to Medicinal Plants of Appalachia* published by the U.S. Department of Agriculture says, "It is also reputed to be an aphrodisiac, particularly for elderly men."

Passionflower was listed as an official plant in the National Formulary from 1916 to 1936 and then fell into disuse. Since 1978 it has been taken off the FDA list of herbs that it recommends as generally safe or effective. By contrast, use of this plant has grown in Europe, and it is a common ingredient in many sedative pharmaceutical products. In Germany, which strictly oversees the use of plants in medicine, it is often combined with valerian in pills.

TEA: Add two to three teaspoons to boiling water, steep, strain and discard the herb. Or add five to ten drops of the tincture to a cup of tranquilizing herbal tea such as catnip, chamomile, lavender, lemon balm or peppermint.

ALERT: Avoid high doses of passionflower during pregnancy.

Rosemary (Rosmarinus officinalis)

Rosemary leaves contain many medicinal properties and the tea has always been thought to be exhilarating and cheering. A primary use of rosemary is to stimulate the nervous system. For a nervous headache that interferes with sleep, drink a tea made of the aerial parts (leaves), or apply warm rosemary tea compresses to the forehead. In the British countryside herbalists make a tincture of rosemary and combine it with small amounts of oats, scullcap or vervain to overcome depression, a frequent cause of insomnia.

Sage (Salvia officinalis)

This common culinary herb literally means "to save." Use it occasionally, singly or added to other aromatic teas, to help with sleep. According to the European folk tradition, sage is useful in lifting depression. The Chinese have imported this herb from Europe for centuries, often exchanging two pounds of their own black tea for one pound of sage. When the sleep of nursing mothers is affected by the weaning process, use sage tea to help dry up the milk.

Valerian (Valerian officinalis)

Valerian is a subtle herb with a delicate, quiet effect. Unlike today's sleeping pills, valerian does not produce grogginess the next day. Peoples of Western Europe have long used the root of *Valerian officinalis* as an effective, safe tranquilizer, pain reliever and sleep inducer. In fact, valerian was so commonly used that it was mentioned often in 19th-century Russian novels and Chekhov plays as a means of sedating overwrought people. Valerian has since been investigated in over 200 scientific papers. Indeed, a Swiss study cited in *Planta Med.* showed that valerian could safely be used for mild insomnia and had few side effects (primarily, it should not be used for long periods or by pregnant women).

The root, aptly called *phu* by the early Greeks, has a strange, almost disagreeable smell. Fortunately, it is available as a tincture, pill and homeopathic pellet as well as in dried root form. Several reliable companies make excellent, but large, valerian pills. I prefer the tiny French discotes (pills) or homeopathic pellets. These can be purchased all over Europe as well as in many health food stores in the United States. I recently purchased a Swiss homeopathic valerian while wandering through the "old city" of Geneva. Sometimes German producers of valerian pills combine it with either melissa or passionflower. Tinctures of valerian are also widely available; use a few drops at a time in tea or a calming bath.

INFUSION: Usually roots have to be simmered in water to make a decoction. But valerian properties are easily released by macerating (steeping) in milk or water. For example, steep three tablespoons of the washed, chopped root in a cup of cold water for half a day. Strain, throw away the root, reserve the liquid, label the jar "Infusion of Valerian Root" and store in the refrigerator. Use small amounts cold, or add several tablespoons to boiling water. To hide the distinctive taste, add drops of peppermint essence or extract, or add the valerian liquid to a strong peppermint, chamomile flower or lemon verbena (melissa) tea. To sweeten, add a teaspoon to a tablespoon of honey. Since honey is also a humectant (a substance which helps the body retain fluid), this may prevent some nighttime awakenings to urinate.

The valerian infusion may also be used in a compress or added to a hot bath to soak away pain and intensify the relaxing action of the hot water. Country doctors of the past had patients bruise valerian root and apply it to their foreheads to relieve headaches.

TINCTURE: Tinctures can be purchased from health food stores, through the mail or you can make your own with small, cleaned chunks of valerian root. If you have a tendency for headaches or allergies, start taking the tincture at half strength, adding eight drops to a cup of cold or boiling water or to a tranquilizing, aromatic tea such as catnip, chamomile, linden or peppermint. Gradually work up to sixteen drops per cup. As a sleep aid, sip a quarter of a cup an hour before going to sleep.

PILLS: I prefer 6c/x homeopathic valerian (you buy them in either 6c or 6x sizes), and I also like the tiny French discotes. With large, nonhomeopathic valerian pills, if you have a tendency for allergy or headaches, test out your reaction by breaking the pill in half.

BATH: To reinforce the sedative action of a long, hot bath and to help assuage anxiety, pain, distress or grief, add up to sixteen drops of the tincture to bathwater.

ALERT: While valerian has been used for centuries and is considered safe, it is not to be used continuously as a nightly sleep potion or if a woman is pregnant. Persistent use, without a break in time, may cause a headache and/or palpitations. Under no circumstances is valerian to be used in combination with a sleeping pill or tranquilizer as it can intensify the action of such drugs.

Homeopathy

Homeopathy is a system of holistic medicine founded in 1790 by the German physician Samuel Hahnemann who discovered the initial concepts of homeopathy during a personal experiment. Dr. Hahnemann was annotating a book of plant medicine and was surprised that Peruvian bark was listed as a cure for malaria because of its astringency. (It is actually the quinine in the bark that is the cure.) He wondered about this because he knew there were many other stronger astringents. As a test he chewed the bark for several days in a row and minutely recorded his reactions. To his astonishment, he quickly developed all the outward symptoms of malaria. When he stopped chewing the bark, the symptoms disappeared. They returned when he chewed the bark again. This led Hahnemann on a unique quest: Could other plant medical cures bring on temporary symptoms of a disease in healthy people? Could that be true of other mineral and animal substances, too? These questions had tremendous implications to the brilliant Hahnemann. It led him to the original concept that like substances could cure like diseases—like cures like.

To evaluate and prove this thesis, Dr. Hahnemann set out with a cadre of healthy volunteers to examine and record their exact reactions to about one hundred natural substances. He called these reactions "provings." Indeed provings was a prophetic word for reactions to substances in healthy people as these reactions "proved" to be primary symptoms of diseases. The natural substance that caused the list of symptoms became the remedy that alleviated or cured the disease.

To protect his healthy subject from such poisonous substances as belladonna or nux vomica, Dr. Hahnemann wisely diluted each product. To his surprise, the greater the dilution of the substance, the stronger its impact. This impelled Dr. Hahnemann to refine his technique, and thereafter all substances were greatly diluted and shaken (succussed).

Examples of how like can cure like are easy to understand with two common substances. When Dr. Hahnemann and his healthy volunteers ingested ground, diluted, unroasted coffee beans (which he called Coffea), they discovered it was a remedy for sleeplessness. Coffee causes insomnia; diluted homeopathic unroasted coffee beans cure insomnia. Another example is the use of honeybee venom (apis) to cure insect stings. Venom in the sting causes a skin reaction, and homeopathic apis relieves the same sting.

Working with his groups of healthy volunteers, Dr. Hahnemann created a vast "picture" of reactions to the one hundred medical substances and drugs. (Several thousand substances have been "proven" since that time.) He then tested these provings on sick people and also added a new dimension in his homeopathic healing technique: an invaluable health and lifestyle questionnaire. Ultimately, he found that the closer the fit of a patient's physical problems and symptoms with the homeopathic substance, the quicker, more effective the cure.

While Dr. Hahnemann had difficulty knowing how or why the system worked, he believed that some subtle form of hidden energy, which he called "vital force," responded to the delicate instigations of the remedies. The natural ability of the body to heal itself then took over and helped rebalance the body. In contrast to the cruel and crude medicine of his time, which included bloodletting, Dr. Hahnemann strongly advised decreasing stress, increasing personal defenses against disease with better hygiene, more bathing and a better diet and tapering down on huge amounts of food, alcohol and coffee used by the general public in his era.

Dr. Hahnemann first published his groundbreaking work, *The Organon of the Rational Art of Healing*, in 1810. Quickly, the system became widely and successfully practiced in Europe, Asia and the United States, especially after homeopaths saved large numbers of patients during a series of decimating epidemics of cholera and the flu. After 1920, homeopathy fell into disuse in the United States, but it continued to be used throughout Europe, especially in England, France and Germany, as well as in India, Sri Lanka, Pakistan and Brazil. In Great Britain, the royal family is under the care of homeopaths. Fortunately, there has been a resurgence of interest in homeopathy in this country as part of the turn toward alternative medicine.

HOMEOPATHIC SLEEP REMEDIES

It is best to use a homeopathic practitioner, but it is possible to use homeopathy if you are careful and attentive to your symptoms. In homeopathy success is achieved by carefully matching the symptoms to the remedy and taking the smallest amount possible for the least amount of time. Never continue remedies if symptoms disappear. Once you have "honed in" on the right remedy, it should work very fast. Experience shows that if the acute problem doesn't get better, you should immediately discontinue the remedy you are using and go on to the next. When the symptoms disappear or improve, discontinue the remedy.

The main homeopathic sleep remedies, each with different symptom matches, are chamomilla, coffea, lycopodium, nux vomica, passiflora (passionflower) and pulsatilla.

- Chamomilla (chamomile) is an exceptional remedy for children, especially when they are unable to sleep because of excitement, pain or irritability. Also use for crying, teething and colic. If possible, purchase in granules.
- Coffea works when you feel a lot of tension, you're too wide awake to fall asleep and if you've drunk too much coffee that day. Use one dose one hour before dinner, and take another dose half an hour before bedtime.
- Lycopodium is the remedy when you cannot fall asleep because you're reviewing the day's events or worrying about what happened during the day. Usually you need this remedy if you cannot sleep most of the night until about daylight and then sleep quite intensely.
- Nux vomica is needed when you overwork, overstudy or drink too much coffee or tea. It is also good when you feel excessively sleepy during the evening time, but after going to bed cannot sleep beyond 2 or 3 A.M.

- Passiflora (passionflower) is recommended when sleep is exceptionally restless and your mind won't stop thinking.
- Pulsatilla works when you are unable to fall asleep early or never before midnight and when you wake again at 3 A.M. Also use when you are awakened and need a snack before getting back to sleep.

HIGHLIGHTS ON HOW TO USE

Homeopathic remedies are usually small lactose (milk sugar) tablets or granules impregnated with what is called the "mother tincture." Here's how a mother tincture of allium is made from onions: The onions are cut, ground, soaked in a closed alcohol/water mixture and succussed (shaken vigorously) for several days. The resulting strained brown liquid is the mother tincture. To make a 1c/x remedy, one drop of the mother tincture is added to 99 drops of alcohol/water mixture and succussed. Each subsequent remedy number is diluted 1:100 [in the decimal form (x), the dilution is 1:10]. So to make a 6x allium, 1/x is diluted by 99 drops and succussed six times.

Each remedy comes named and with a number. The number denotes how much the remedy has been diluted from the mother tincture. In homeopathy, the higher number is the one diluted the most. Paradoxically, the more the substance is diluted, the stronger it becomes. Note that you can buy remedies in *either* c or x sizes, which are abbreviated here as c/x.

Lactose pills come in tablet, pillule, powder and granule form. Pillules are the tiny pills usually found in family homeopathic kits (such kits are available by mail order; one source is Homeopathic Educational Services, listed in the Resources). One tablet or pillule is the dose for adult or child. Granules, although less available, are easier for infants and children to use simply because they dissolve more easily and are therefore harder to spit out. It is permissable to dissolve a remedy in a six-ounce glass of water and take two teaspoons at suggested intervals. There is also a liquid solution for those who are lactose allergic (two drops on the tongue for an adult, one drop for a child). Take between meals or at least a half hour before eating. Rinse mouth out before taking.

DOSAGES VARY FOR DIFFERENT CONDITIONS:

- Chronic (long-standing) insomnia or other disorders: Use 6c/x.
- Acute condition or emergency: Normally take two tablets of 6c/x every two to four hours. However, for a high fever, headache, lengthy, intense crying or a sudden assault of insomnia, you can use a higher potency, usually a 30c/x. Take one dose every fifteen minutes for one

hour. If you see no change after four doses, or one hour, it is not the right remedy. Try another suggested remedy.

- Nonacute condition: For a normal illness such as the beginning of a cold, earache or sore throat (usually not a sleep situation), take one dose every two hours. If your nose stops running, your ear appears not to hurt or your throat isn't as sore, the remedy is working, and you can cut back on the dose. Thereafter, use three times a day.
- Children (newborn to teens): Unless advised otherwise, it is safer for children to take lower-numbered remedies from 3c/x, 6c/x, 9c/x to 12c/x.
- Infants: Dissolve one granule or pellet in cool water, draw up the liquid in a clean eyedropper and give warm under the tongue or in a bottle of water. If using granules, use just enough to cover tiny area of small fingernail or a small pinch. If using liquid homeopathic remedy, dissolve in warm water to get rid of alcohol base.
- Toddlers and older: Drop one granule or pellet onto a clean spoon and deposit under the child's tongue. Tell the child not to chew, but allow the pellet to dissolve under the tongue. (When administering, adults should wash their hands and avoid touching the pellets.) When the child's symptoms improve, stop the remedy (unless a repeat dose is suggested). If by chance symptoms are aggravated in any way, stop the remedy immediately and try another.
- Caution: When using homeopathic remedies, homeopaths advise avoiding contamination with asprin, laxatives, sleeping pills, nasal drops, liniments, camphor (Chap Stick), patent medicines of any kind or strong smelling food substances such as peppermint, caffeine or caffeine-loaded soft drinks since these interfere with the effect of the remedy. Store remedies in an airtight, clean, dry, cool, dark place.

Tissue Salts

Tissue salts, also called cell salts, are easy-to-use, effective and safe natural remedies. Though they have been used since the 1800s, they are not widely known by the American public. The system of tissue salts was developed in 1873 by a German homeopathic physician, Dr. William Schuessler. (Often tissue or cell salts are called Schuessler salts.) Over the course of many experiments Dr. Schuessler found that many diseases as well as negative mind states occurred when a patient became deficient in certain inorganic minerals. He determined there were twelve such minerals (salts) and they were all essential to the proper growth and development of the human body. As a homeopath, Dr. Schuessler concluded that each deficiency brought on specific symptoms.

Like Dr. Hahnemann, Dr. Schuessler "proved" his symptom picture on healthy volunteers. Then he gave specific minerals to sick patients according to his symptom picture for each mineral. Dr. Schuessler found that once a missing mineral is replaced, the body readjusts and heals itself. He also emphasized that tissue salts should not be thought of as a cure, but rather a remedy that could overcome a deficiency.

TISSUE SALT SLEEP AIDS

Tissue salts that aid sleep include the following:

- Kali Phos. (potassium phosphate) is a nerve and brain nutrient found in all tissues of the body. Essential for metabolism, it is the main tissue remedy for sleeplessness, especially when that stems from over-excitement, brain fatigue or overwork. It is also indicated for sleep-walking. It should be used with other salts if the condition is chronic. Kali Phos. is needed when one has symptoms of irritability, depression and frequent urination. Use this tissue salt for periods of weariness, continual periods of yawning or needing to stretch. Also, use Kali Phos. for nighttime twitching and children's night terrors (when they wake up screaming from a sound sleep). This is the mineral to use when one has frightening dreams of fire, ghosts, falling or robbers.
- Natrum Mur. (sodium chloride) controls the ebb and flow of bodily fluids and is wonderfully useful when one awakes unrefreshed from sleep. Nat. Mur. is the appropriate remedy if one has consistent fatigue upon awakening in the morning or if one has a constant desire to sleep. Use it when one is too restless to fall asleep, especially if that is coupled with a feeling that the legs are cold. It is also useful when one resists sleep until very late in the evening and for leg starts.
- Natrum Sulph. (sodium sulphate) should be used when one is awakened by asthma.
- Calcarea Fluor (calcium fluoride) is the remedy for dreams that are extremely vivid. Dreams might include new scenes and places or a sense of impending danger or death.
- Calcarea Phos. (calcium phosphate) is the remedy for children who cry out at night, who are hard to wake in the morning and who constantly stretch and yawn. It is also good for periods of excessive drowsiness in elderly people.
- Magnesia Phos. (magnesium phosphate) is used for insomnia caused

by strong emotional states and nervousness. It can be used when sleep is elusive because of exhaustion or the brain is tired.

- Natrum Phos. (sodium phosphate) should be used when sleeplessness is involved with digestive disturbances or if one is very drowsy yet cannot sleep.
- Kali Mur. (potassium chloride) is used for restless sleep and when one is startled by the least noise.
- Ferrum Phos. (iron phosphate) is the oxygen carrier and is a vital adjunct to any other treatment, no matter what the symptoms. It is used for those who are drowsy in the afternoon and restless at night and have anxious dreams.
- A combination of all twelve salts is also available. Many nutritionists advise using it on a daily basis as a mineral supplement.

Specific tissue salts are listed in the At-a-Glance Charts in Chapters 4 through 6 for several dozen problems and symptoms related to sleep-lessness, including bedwetting, dreaming, drowsiness, exclamations during dreams, headaches, heavy or anxious dreams, incontinence, irritability, jerking limbs during sleep, nightmares, noises in the head, screaming in sleep, sleepiness, sleepwalking, teething, twitching, and wakefulness.

As with homeopathy, the inorganic salts are greatly diluted. If you can find 1c or 1x, 2c or 2x or 3c or 3x, use them for children, but most homeopaths successfully use 6c or 6x tissue salts for all remedies.

HOW TO TAKE TISSUE SALTS

It is best not to contaminate tissue salts, which come in tiny pellets, by touching them with your hands. Shake them directly under the tongue and let them dissolve.

DOSAGES:

- The average adult dose is five tissue salts.
- The dose for an infant is one tissue salt. You can dissolve the tablet in a little warm water and feed it, when cool, to the child in an eye dropper.
- The dose for toddlers and older children is two tissue salts. Shake out two tablets onto a clean spoon and place them under the child's tongue. Be sure to tell the child not to chew them, but to let them dissolve.

FREQUENCY: Take tissue salts at the following intervals according to the seriousness of the problem:

- Acute: One dose every ten minutes. For extra impact, dissolve the pellets in a little hot water. As soon as there is some relief, cut back.
- Less acute: One dose every two hours.
- Chronic cases: Three doses a day.
- When two tissue salts are suggested: Take an alternate dose of each salt. In an acute case take the first remedy on the hour and the second remedy on the half hour. In nonacute cases, alternate the tissue salt therapy at the even hour.

Bach Flower Remedies

Dr. Edward Bach was an eminent bacteriologist and surgeon who practiced on famed Harley Street in London at the early part of this century. After reading Dr. Hahnemann's book, he gradually turned his practice over to homeopathy. In observing his patients, Dr. Bach decided that many of their illnesses were a result of their fears and negative moods and attitudes. After much thought, he decided there were twelve states of mind: fear, terror, mental torture and worry, indecision, indifference or boredom, doubt or discouragement, overconcern, weakness, self-distress, impatience, overenthusiasm, pride or aloofness. He believed that if patients could over-come these negative emotions, it would help them thwart potential illnesses.

Dr. Bach was inspired to discover flower remedies prepared in the ho-meopathic fashion which could overcome these negative emotions. Through a profound process of observation and experimentation through the fields, meadows and woods of Britain, Dr. Bach eventually found 38 flower remedies, which he infused from pure flowers on dew in the sun. He also created one overview remedy which he brilliantly named "Rescue Remedy." It does just that. It pulls people out of crying jags, helps them after a trauma, perks them up and tones down upsets of all kinds. You can purchase these remedies and books about Dr. Bach's system in most health food stores.

The best Bach flower remedies for different types of sleep problems:

- Rescue Remedy seems to work in almost any situation, especially when you need to calm down.
- Being angry can destroy sleep, and Holly is the Bach remedy recom-mended for such a state.

- Everyone at some time has "pit-bull" thoughts, the kind that just won't let go and insist on invading your mind. They go around and around as if on a merry-go-round. To offset persistent worrying thoughts, turn to White Chestnut.
- Caregivers can try Hornbeam or Olive when they need some inner help to get a job done or when you feel squeezed about the amount of work you have to do.
- Larch is for confidence. Take it when you have doubts about your ability or if you are wondering if you are capable of doing the job ahead.
- When schedules and tasks make one feel spacey and unable to concentrate, take Clematis.
- For periods of resentfulness and bitterness, take Willow.
- For depression and gloom, take Mustard Flower.
- If you are a person who tends to hide worries under a cloak of cheerfulness and good humor, take Agrimony.
- There are a wide variety of remedies for depression, thoughts about death, obsessions with others and fears of various kinds.

9

Water: An Ideal Aid to Sleep

Water is one of the world's primal natural remedies. In its many temperatures and forms—liquid, steam and ice—water provides a wide range of safe, inexpensive home treatments that promote sleep. A flick of the faucet provides either hot or cold running water for direct application to the body. The freezer provides instant access to anti-pain ice or chemical cold packs. It is a simple task to boil water for sleep-encouraging herbal teas or to produce enough steam to overcome nasal congestion. Cloths dipped into herbal teas and positioned on stiff or cramped muscles relax areas thwarting sleep. The variety of water treatments described here should prove surprising and useful.

How do external water treatments lull reluctant humans into sleep? Water treatments, whether hot or cold, generate a subtle change in energy by compelling new patterns of circulation. Hot and tepid water baths are helpful in inducing sleep because they totally relax the mind and the body. Hot full baths are a form of passive heat, which first slightly raises, then gradually lowers body temperature. This promotes sleep in an indirect way. As soon as our temperature drops, we are designed by nature to feel slightly drowsy and therefore more ready for sleep. A partial hot bath directed to the feet invites sleep by diverting blood from the head to the feet and the trunk. This temporarily lowers brain activity and mimics the normally languid state of presleep.

Cold water applications work differently, but also use the skin's physiological programming to advantage. One of the skin's main functions is to maintain a certain temperature. When cold water is applied externally, the body responds by sending fresh reserves of blood to the area that has been deliberately cooled. The blood rushes to the area and heats the area from within. This physiological reaction can be used to encourage sleep, as well as for a host of other health needs.

Hot and Cold Water Therapies

The water treatments that can coax one into a tranquil presleep state include warm sponging, lukewarm (neutral) or full hot baths, hot foot baths, hot, moist head and spinal compresses, cold stocking compresses and the cold abdominal compress called "Neptune's Girdle." Cold water massages are further aids. For long-term revitalization, try cold water treading.

One inevitably feels refreshed after a bath and friction rub, and this helps most people fall asleep more quickly. This is particularly true of children. Unfortunately, adult insomniacs carry a lifetime of delaying tactics with them to their bed. People who are chronically sleepless should reinforce water therapy by practicing "sleep mindfulness," a presleep awareness that alerts the mind and the body that it is time to go to sleep. To intensify that languid state, use any of the physical and mental exercises described in Chapter 10.

WARM SPONGE BATH

This is the simplest of all the friction baths and can be used for insomnia, especially for children, fevered states and weak patients who need to sleep.

After changing the bed linens and drawing the blinds or curtains, splash the face with warm water and dry. Keep the body enveloped in a light cotton blanket or a large towel and only expose one small section at a time while sponging it. Use a large, soft sponge and dip it into either warm water or warm water laced with apple cider vinegar (use a quarter cup of apple cider vinegar to a cup of plain water). Rub each section of the body vigorously, moving from the upper to the lower part. After thoroughly drying your body and putting on nightclothes, turn out all the lights and go to bed with a light blanket covering your body. This should produce a restful sleep.

NEUTRAL BATH

Anyone in any stage of health can take a fifteen-minute neutral temperature (the same temperature as the body) bath. Be sure to keep the room free of drafts, and prevent a feeling of chilliness by covering the chest and the back with a hotter, moist towel. To deepen the relaxation of any warm or hot bath, make your neck and therefore the rest of your body more comfortable in the bathtub with a rubber pillow or rolled towel. By tradition such baths calm and sedate the body, relaxing muscles and easing bones. Gently towel dry and go to bed immediately. To overcome great fatigue, add to the bathwater a cup of apple cider vinegar, a cup of coarse salt or some essence of pine.

FULL HOT BATH

Most people turn instinctively to a long, hot bath when they are overtired, have overexercised or feel on the verge of a cold. In general, immersion in hot water acts like a sedative. The action of the heat and the body's natural counteraction produce total relaxation and calm.

Start running the bath at body temperature or slightly higher, get into the bath and gradually increase the water temperature until it is as high as the body can tolerate. This is the time to add one or several aromatic herbs or minerals.

- Some examples are aromatic and relaxing extract of pine or drops of lavender oil.
- To reduce agitation or a worried state, add a few drops of calming valerian extract or chamomile tea or extract. Capsules in various sizes from many European sources are available in health food stores.
- Epsom salts, available in drug stores, are another choice. Add a half cup to a cup of Epsom salts to the bath. Epsom salt baths are very powerful, and because they produce profuse perspiration, the bath acts to detoxify the body. The heat of the water and the action of the dissolved salts are depleting and will produce a lethargy and drowsiness. For this reason, never take this bath unless you are prepared to go right to sleep. And do not take this or any very hot bath if you are very young, very old, pregnant, have heart trouble, are ill with a chronic disease or are in a weakened state.

Remain in the bath from two to twenty minutes depending on your comfort and need. Before you get out of a hot bath, slowly drizzle cool water into the hot mix. (As a general rule, it's best to end all hot baths and showers with slightly cooler water to offset the depleting effect of the hot water.) Get out and towel dry. If you are very desirous of instant sleep, wrap yourself in a large bath sheet, and pop right into bed enveloped in it. Cover yourself with your favorite blanket or down cover. You will feel cozy and warm within seconds, and this helps ensure drowsiness. Allow yourself to quietly doze off into a profound and peaceful sleep.

Sleep researchers have studied the effect of passive heat from hot baths, noting that the bath has special success if taken several hours before bedtime. This gives the body time to let the initial rise in temperature become slightly lower. As the temperature goes down, drowsiness inevitably sets in.

HOT FOOT BATH

A hot foot bath temporarily draws blood from the head region and makes one drowsy. For several minutes dip both your feet into several inches of moderately hot water. Dry your feet and go right to bed. If you are also trying to overcome a bad cold or cough, add mustard powder to the water. (See Resources for Dr. Singha's Bath.)

HOT, MOIST COMPRESSES

To encourage a feeling of drowsiness, apply a hot, moist compress to the head for a few minutes. (A compress is a cloth dipped into either hot water or a hot herbal tea; see Chapter 8 for more about compresses.) The same drowsiness can be produced by applying a series of short (up to five minutes) hot compresses to the lower spine. Replace the compress as soon as it cools off.

COLD, WET SOCK COMPRESS

This cold compress ends up heating the body. An old-country remedy, it relaxes the body, overcomes exhaustion and produces a quiet sleep. When the cold, wet compress is applied to the feet, the body acts to warm the feet immediately and temporarily sends blood from other areas of the body, including the head, to heat up the feet. As soon as the head is decongested and blood flows elsewhere, drowsiness sets in. Note that this same technique may be used to decongest a head cold.

Dip knee-high cotton socks into cold water or apple cider vinegar and water. Wring out. Apply immediately to each foot. Completely cover the wet area with long woolen socks. If no long cotton socks are available, use strips of cotton. If no long woolen socks or scarves are available, make the area airtight by covering with strips of plastic wrap or brown paper. The compress takes about an hour or two to become effective, but it may be left on all night to produce relaxed sleep.

COLD DOUBLE ABDOMINAL COMPRESS/
NEPTUNE'S GIRDLE

This cold abdominal pack, also known as "Neptune's Girdle," is a complicated compress, which has been continually praised over the 150 years of hydrotherapy. It generally exhibits complex and remarkable results in sedation, and when used over a course of time, it helps overcome chronic insomnia. A series of these applications also acts to tone the digestive organs. Neptune's Girdle is one of several instances where cold (in this case not too cold, but tepid) applications produce heating effects.

In a warm room without drafts apply a large wet, tepid or cold compress to the abdomen, using about three yards of light, coarse toweling. Wet about half the toweling in tepid water and wring out. Apply to the abdomen, wrapping around front and back, so that there are at least two layers of thickness. Wind the rest of the dry cloth snugly around the abdomen and back. Fasten with safety pins or a thin cord. Cover the entire wet area with a larger dry flannel cloth that is airtight. Fasten and leave on the entire night.

The body reacts internally to this cold application by immediately sending large amounts of blood to heat the area and normalize its temperature. This diverts a substantial portion of the body's blood to the trunk, causing a temporary contraction of the cerebral blood vessels and producing an immediate drowsiness. A tranquilizing effect sets in almost at once. Discontinue the pack if a chill sets in for any reason.

Note that this compress can be used to treat chronic digestive problems and a high fever. With a fever, change the compress every thirty minutes— about the time the cloth takes to dry completely. Wash your abdomen with cool water, and dry with light strokes. Repeat several times until your fever comes down. (The following cold mitten massage is another easy, effective fever reduction technique.)

COLD MITTEN MASSAGE

This is a refreshing, stimulating massage which helps build resistance to disease, overcome fevers and promote good circulation in the body, all of which enhance the sleep process.

Cover your body with a large towel. Wet a washcloth or a soft fiber mitten under cold water or a mixture of cold water and apple cider vinegar, and wring it out. Expose one section of your body at a time, preferably starting with your upper torso and shoulders. Rub the section vigorously. Dry the area, cover it, and move on to another part of the body, until you have massaged your whole body.

SALT RUB

A wonderful tonic, this massage is exhilarating and refreshing to the system. It helps overcome fatigue and promotes relaxation as it stimulates the body. It can be done immediately before bed, but, if done one to several hours before sleep, it has an even stronger impact by bracing, energizing and preparing the body for peaceful sleep.

This rub is most easily done in a full bath, but it can also be done in a shower. Purchase a supply of coarse Kosher salt, the kind so beloved of great cooks. Pour some into your hand, and rub it all over your shoulders, arms and torso. Then massage your thighs, knees and feet, including the bottoms.

COLD WATER TREADING

Each day you practice treading in cold water will bring more vitality and good health into your life. The reason it is called "treading" is because the hydrotherapists who developed it had their patients walking or marching in water. If you're doing it in a bathtub or shower, it helps to hold on to something, preferably a wall grip. Treading can also be done sitting down on a stool in the bathtub and marching in place.

Start this revitalization program by dipping your toes under cold running water in your bathtub for thirty seconds or so. If you only have a shower, end a warm to hot shower with a burst of cold water on your feet. Gradually increase the time of each cold application; eventually you will enjoy the cold. Your first goal can be a few-second to one-minute application. Then increase the time until you are happy with at least a three-to-five-minute period of cold water immersion. If you are doing this with children, make sure to start out very slowly and have them hold on to your hand or a wall grip.

At-a-Glance Chart of Water Therapies

For a discussion of how each therapy works physiologically, see the text.

SLEEP PROBLEM	WATER THERAPIES	OTHER FACTS OF INTEREST
Chronic insomnia	• Drink sedative teas daily in the early part of the day. • Take leisurely *full hot bath*. • Immerse feet in shallow *hot foot bath*. • Series of three *hot, moist compresses* to lower spine. • Occasionally apply *Neptune's Girdle*.	• Eliminate coffee and regular (caffeinated) tea. • Practice sleep mindfulness (Chapter 10). • Caution: Do not take a full hot bath if your are pregnant, chronically ill, very old, very young or have any indication of heart trouble.
Chronic and occasional insomnia	Long-range revitalization techniques: • Daily *treading in cold water*. • *Friction rubs* with cold wet crocheted mitten or course salt. • Series or occasional use of *Neptune's Girdle*.	
Mild case of sleeplessness	• Apply *hot moist compress to head* for a few minutes. • Take *hot foot bath* for a few minutes.	
Tired: Need a good night's sleep	• Take a 15-minute *neutral bath*. • Take a sedative *full hot bath*.	• Optional: Add herbal essences or Epsom Salts.

SLEEP PROBLEM	WATER THERAPIES	OTHER FACTS OF INTEREST
Sleeplessness due to too much studying or thinking	To relieve head congestion: • Take brief *hot foot bath*. Occasionally follow with tonic alternating hot and cold stream of water to the bottom of the feet. • Apply sedative *cold wet stockings*.	
Awakened during the night: Cannot go back to sleep	Two to three times a week immerse the lower part of the body in a shallow (only a few inches of water) sitz bath.	

Physical and Mental Exercises

Being able to fall effortlessly into refreshing and restorative sleep has long been associated with a healthy balance of mind and body. In fact, sleep specialists recommend a well-rounded program of physical exercise and overall fitness as the first avenue to ensuring a good night's sleep. The many physical and mental exercises in this chapter, which have been culled from a wide variety of sources, are all designed to help you get the sleep you need to live life to the fullest.

Physical Exercises

Nothing helps induce restful, healthy sleep like regular exercise. When the body feels toned and alert, sleep is much easier and instantaneous. The only caveat is to avoid serious or vigorous exercise just before bedtime. Stretching each part of the body combined with relaxation imagery, "thinking darkness" with warmed palms, deep and subtle breathing, alternate nostril breathing and mind-stretching exercises are all very helpful in inducing sleep. Some gentle and appropriate sleep-inducing exercises follow. Most of these easy concepts can also be practiced by youngsters.

REGULAR EXERCISE

After only fifteen minutes of an exercise, whether it be walking, swimming, biking or line dancing, the body produces chemical endorphins which helps lift away despair and gloom. A recent report from the Surgeon General advocates moderate exercise not only to control weight but to dramatically reduce the risk of potential health (and sleep) disorders created by high blood pressure, diabetes type 2 and gastrointestinal and cardiovascular problems.

To overcome insomnia, find something you like to do to keep you moving and do it three to five times a week. The exercise can be fast social dancing for a half an hour, pushing a stroller one and a half miles in a half hour, washing and waxing a car for three quarters of an hour to an hour, washing windows or floors for three quarters of an hour to an hour or playing basketball for as little as fifteen minutes.

Depression often causes insomnia, and one of the best ways to lift depression is with exercise. A writer friend, who was once fond of saying, "Whenever I feel like exercising, I lie down until the feeling goes away," moved from the East to sunny California. He recently confided, "I feel like another person. I am another person. In my past life I was depressed every day. But here we have a pool, so I began to swim each day. I liked my neighbors, and since they played tennis several times a week, I took lessons in order to play with them. My insomnia and my depression evaporated! I'm never depressed anymore." My friend discovered the fountain of youth and one of the best cures for insomnia and depression.

BREATHING EXERCISES

Since oxygen is vital to every cell in your body, the way you breathe can influence the way your entire body functions, including the way you sleep. Given the many stresses of everyday life, most Americans don't breathe deeply enough. When was the last time you took a really deep breath? Making contact with your body through your breath is an important way of reconnecting with yourself. It will also ensure you get a better night's sleep.

Breathe Deeply
Each night as you are preparing to go to bed—even as you are doing your last chores, watching your favorite TV show or taking your bath or shower—concentrate your mind and body by turning your attention to your breath. Breathe as deeply as possible. Turn aside all other thoughts, worries and problems of the day.

In addition to rhythmic deep breathing, also go in your mind's eye to a beautiful place that you can recall. It can be a place you have visited or a recollection of a beautiful scene you have seen in a photograph. Chances are it will be outdoors and near some water, maybe a beach by the sea, a lagoon or a stream that you canoed as a child. Perhaps it will be a mountain village. Keep it simple. Visualize this glorious place, all the while focusing on your breath. Keep thinking, breathing and remembering this exquisite, harmonious place. Envision yourself there in that place, happy, healthy and serene. Practice this exercise whenever you feel tense and as often as you can before sleep. Add a yawn or two to this exercise for extra help in getting to sleep.

Whenever you are tense, practice deep, concentrated breathing. This will relax you instantly. One of the best relaxation techniques is to close your eyes, breathe deeply and count backwards from ten to one. This slows down the whole body and makes it receptive to any imagination exercises.

Breathing and Imagining

A mental writing exercise that brings on sleep is writing the number 3 over and over again. There is something hypnotic about the curves of the 3, and fairly soon the mind feels exhausted and ready for sleep.

Imagine you are standing at a large school blackboard. Take a piece of chalk and write down the number 3. Erase it. Write down 3 again. Erase it. Write down 3 again. Something about the curves in the 3 gets harder and harder to write. As you get sleepier and sleepier, don't resist oncoming sleep. Give in to it. Yawn, yawn again. Keep on writing and erasing those 3s until sleep overtakes you.

I also like this slightly harder variation. In your mind, count backwards from ten to one. Imagine you are at a school blackboard. Pick up a piece of chalk in your dominant hand and see yourself writing the number 100 on the blackboard. Mentally take an eraser, erase the number and write 99. Erase the 99. Put down the eraser. Take up the chalk and again see yourself writing the number 98. Keep on erasing and writing the numbers backwards from 100 as far as you have to before falling asleep. A tremendous effort seems to be involved in "grabbing" the numbers backward. As you get sleepier and sleepier, don't resist oncoming sleep. Give in to it.

Bottle Breathing

Eleanor Tomic of Montara, California, does this breathing and imaging inhalation every night and says it never fails to put her to sleep. It may help your visualization if you imagine you are filling a bottle with water. What fills up first? The bottom of the bottle. Keep that image in mind because as you breathe in air, you will be filling the bottom of your body—your abdomen and diaphragm (not your chest).

- Inhale, letting air flow deeply into your abdominal center. Extend your belly outward and exaggerate the extension.
- Immediately pinch your nose closed, to hold your breath.
- Without delay, let the air in your belly move up to your chest (your belly will flatten).

- Then, still holding your nose, shift air back into your belly and repeat the shift again to your chest.
- Release your nose and breathe normally.

"This makes me feel calm and as if I have been massaged internally," says Tomic. She advises people to experiment and adapt this exercise to their own abilities and needs.

Drop Your Jaw and Yawn

We all know how catching a yawn is. One person does it, and soon everyone in the room is yawning. It comes from the need for more oxygen. I learned the value of a yawn and its effect on sleep when I was a teenager.

The occasion was a beautiful night on Lake George. A group of us had canoed from our island camp site to see the sunset on Commission Island, the northern-most camping island on the lake. The sunset was fine, but soon a fearsome storm arose with torrential rain, thunder and threatening lightning. Fortunately, we all had our sleeping bags and decided to stay on the island. But I couldn't fall asleep. As I tossed and turned in my sleeping bag, our leader grumbled: "Lie still, drop your jaw and just yawn! Yawn a few times!" I did and I fell asleep instantly. That's when I discovered yawning is better than any sleeping pill and works even when you're tired and can't fall asleep.

I later learned from yogi practitioners that yawning can be reinforced by holding the tongue behind the lower teeth. If one is a long-term insomniac, it may take several nights of vigorous, intentional yawning to break through old "can't-sleep" barriers. The trick is to keep trying.

RELAXING EXERCISES AND STRETCHES

The following exercises and stretches are specifically designed to relax and balance every part of your body, encouraging it to fall naturally into a sound and refreshing sleep. Practice them routinely or whenever you're stressed.

Relax Your Eyes

Tension and fatigue in the eyes can influence the speed with which you fall asleep. In fact, if your eyes are so tense and tired, you don't think you can sleep, palming your eyes just before going to sleep will completely relax them. Vigorously rub your palms together for a few minutes, and place them over your eyes. Keep your eyes closed and enjoy the total blackness of the palming. This technique, also called "thinking darkness," can be done at any time during the day to relax tired eyes.

The Elephant Swing

The eminent natural medicine interpreter Dr. Marsh Morrison was a friend of my father. Among the many relaxing things Dr. Morrison shared with us was his elephant swing that takes away tension from the eyes.

To practice the elephant swing, stand with your feet apart. Loosen up by gently shaking your arms, head and feet. With your head slightly downwards and your eyes open and not staring, let your arms hang loosely by your sides. Then bring them up together in wide arcs, as if you were an elephant swinging his trunk. Blink your eyes whenever you feel like it; this enhances eye relaxation. Do these swings for several minutes. You'll soon find you're relaxed and ready for bed.

Bottoms Up Like a Baby

Kneel on a mat or carpet, sitting back on your legs, and stretch your body and face forward until your head touches the floor. Stay there as comfortably as possible. While this position may not sound comfortable, it is totally relaxing. In fact, you will be duplicating the posture of a baby: your backside will be up in the air, your head gently leaning on the floor, your hands stretched forward. Stay there for three to five minutes, feeling completely relaxed. Some experts advise resting your head on flat, folded blankets.

Older people may find it easier to do this exercise at a table or desk. Place about five folded blankets at one end of the surface, and stretch your upper torso over the blankets. Reach your arms forward, or hold them comfortably around your head and neck. This stretch relieves all the tension in the upper shoulders and neck.

Body Alignment Stretch

While I was in England, I discovered this reposturing tip that helps keep the body aligned, prevents fatigue and encourages proper positioning while sleeping. It can be done many times during the day. Stand against a wall, with your feet about six inches apart and your heels touching the wall. Make sure your hips, shoulders and head are touching the wall. Walk away from the wall in that same tall posture.

Neck Stretch

Most people carry their tension in their neck and shoulders. That's why it's important to relax one's neck before going to bed. This exercise is best done standing or sitting with closed eyes. Softly lower the neck downwards. Gently roll the neck in a circle, upwards to the right, backwards and then downwards to the left. Keep making gentle circles to stretch and relax the muscles of the neck. Then reverse directions. This can be done any time of the day.

Shoulder Stretch

If your shoulders are tense from reading or sitting too long, stretch your shoulders to relax them. Take a deep breath, hold the breath and raise your right shoulder. Lift it, roll it forward and around in a circle. Exhale. Repeat with the left shoulder.

Arm Stretch

While either standing or sitting, take a deep breath and raise your arms to shoulder height. Stretch your fingers. Make believe your fingers are airborne and you are flying away.

Relaxing Lower Back Stretch

This lifting stretch can be done before sleep lying either on the floor or on your bed. It is an incredibly restful and relaxing position, and it works like a charm, even if you only do it for a few minutes. However, the best stretch takes about ten to fifteen minutes.

Lie down on the floor, raise your lower legs and thighs up and rest your knees and your feet on a chair, bed or sofa. Put your arms gently out to your sides so they are limp and relaxed. Your back and head should be completely on the ground. (You end up in a square-shaped S position.) Stretch your neck so it doesn't feel cramped, and yawn a bit. If you wish, you can make your head more comfortable by supporting it with a small rolled towel under your neck. You'll find lower back pain disappears as if by magic. If you find the floor too hard or you feel uncomfortable doing this, lie on a mat or use two long towels folded lengthwise to support your spine.

The Shake That Improves Sleep

My father has been proved right countless times with this age-old instruction: "If you are tense and you need to relax the body, shake your ankles!" Strange as it sounds, when the ankles are at ease, the rest of the body becomes calmer. Just before bed, shake your ankles and jiggle your toes.

Antigravity Leg Exercise

Many of us who have been working hard or walking or standing too much sometimes feel bone tired, but too tired to sleep. Here's an exercise that flushes acid wastes from the leg muscles and helps promote sleep.

- Lie on your back on the floor with your hips propped against an arm chair or sofa and your bare feet stretched towards the ceiling.
- Let go completely so that your ankles and feet are limp.
- From your thighs, vigorously jiggle your legs, ankles and feet for twenty seconds.
- Reach up with two hands to your right ankle and press ("milk") it gently. Move your hands downwards from your ankle to your foot and then from your ankle up your thighs, pressing each inch along the way. Relax your right foot.
- Jiggle your left foot and repeat the inch-by-inch pressing, finally relaxing your left foot.

Sleep Pressure Points

Thousands of years ago the Chinese discovered points on the body that could prevent illness and remedy most health situations. They developed a method of stimulating these points with slender, hair-like needles that is called "acupuncture." There are several offshoots of this system: martial arts pressure points, Japanese finger pressure points called "shiatsu" and Chinese pressure points called "acupressure." In Asia the following points have been successfully used to promote sleep.

Hand

The Shen-man point is the most important pressure point for sleep. With your hand facing you, locate the point at the outside of the wrist crease, below the pinky finger. Use your thumb to press hard for fifteen to twenty seconds on one and then the other wrist.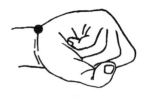

The Self Care Catalog sells an excellent acupressure device for the Shen-man point: a little metal nipple that is attached with self-adhesive (see Resources).

Neck

The An-mien point is one inch below the bottom of your ear lobe. Use your index finger to press hard for fifteen to twenty seconds on one side and then the other side of your neck.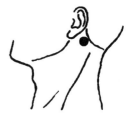

Breastbone
Press deeply for ten seconds on the center of your breastbone in line with the nipples.

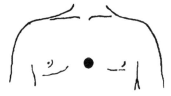

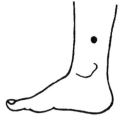

Leg
The San-yin-chiao point is three inches above your ankle bone on the inside of your calf. Use your thumb and press hard for five to ten seconds on one and then the other calf.

Toes

- On the big toe, find the point on the lower corner of the nail on the side nearest the other toes, and press hard for five or ten seconds on one and then the other toe.
- On the fourth toe, find the point on the lower corner of the nail on the side nearest the small toe, and press hard for five to ten seconds on one and then the other toe.

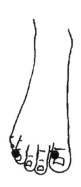

Finger Holding to "Let Go"
I learned this Asian letting-go technique from a Chinese friend. Just as you are going to sleep gently wrap and cradle each finger for several minutes; use the opposite hand to delicately create a mold around each finger. Start by cradling the thumb first, then do all the other fingers. Do both hands.

Special Points for Children

- A general point to relax and pacify an irritable child at any point during the day or night is at the "third eye" between the eyebrows. Press it gently with your thumb for five to ten seconds.
- The big toe point also helps children sleep.
- For teething problems, the Ho-ku point is the most valuable. Place your thumb or index finger at the edge of the webbing between the baby's thumb and index finger. Gently press for about five to ten seconds on one and then the other hand.

- Another toothache point is on the back of the baby's ankle parallel to the ankle bone. Gently press the point for about ten seconds on one and then the other ankle.

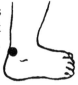

Mental Exercises

People are becoming increasingly aware of the integral connection between mind and body. The following mental exercises will enable you to get to sleep more easily and sleep without recurring nightmares. One exercise will even help you tap your problem-solving capabilities while you are sleeping.

Sleep Mindfulness
Sleep mindfulness is a presleep awareness that alerts the mind and the body that it is time to go to sleep. It works best if you make up your own brief script, including such phrases as "I am going to sleep now. I anticipate falling asleep quickly and pleasurably. I will stay asleep. If I wake up during the night, I plan to go back to sleep immediately." During sleep mindfulness, accept the act of going to sleep and will your thoughts to wander through to a pleasant, euphoric state. Do not allow any distracting activities, such as telephone calls, reading in bed, listening to the radio or watching TV during this period.

Stop Recurrent Nightmares with Constructive Dreaming Techniques
Constructive dreaming is an exciting and successful technique which can help you rethink difficulties, change priorities and reestablish new personal strategies for every part of your life, including your sleeping time.

One of the best uses for constructive dreaming techniques is to stop recurrent nightmares. For instance, just before you go to bed, write down the recurring nightmare in clear, concise words. An example of a recurring nightmare is finding yourself naked in front of an audience; another concerns teeth falling out; yet another is almost drowning in white water and being unable to reach the shore. Think about it for a while, and then write down how you would ideally change the nightmare so it wouldn't be a nightmare anymore. Tell yourself, "From now on, this will be the dream I have, and this is the ending I want."

One young woman I know had a fear of being followed by a rapist. She rethought her nightmare and "instructed" her presleep mind that she no longer wanted that dream to occur. "I want to be in control of my life," she told herself. "I want to turn around and confront this person who is following me and demand that they stop!" She did just that, and the dream never came back. Further, she realized the dream wasn't so much about a rapist following her as it was about her seizing control of the chaotic parts of her life. When she started thinking about that problem, she was able to work out many new strategies for a successful lifestyle.

Harness Your Dreaming Mind with Presleep Questions
Most scientists use their dreaming mind to produce possible solutions to the problems they are working on. One celebrated solution to a knotty chemical problem, the shape of the carbon ring of benzene, occurred to the famed German chemist, Friedrich August Kekulé, during a dream. He dreamt he saw six snakes swallowing their own tails. When he awakened, he instantly understood the dream's meaning: the shape was a hexagon! Science historians tell us this was "the most brilliant prediction found in the range of organic chemistry," which is of fundamental importance to modern chemistry.

Dr. Roger Williams, the innovative researcher who discovered the B-complex vitamin pantothenic acid, practiced his own version of dream therapy. Just before going to bed Williams would think about his problem. When he awakened during the night, he would get out of bed and sit in the dark, thinking about his problem from different vantage points. Fifteen minutes to an hour later, he went back to bed with the problem fresh in his brain. His sleeping (creative) brain arranged, organized and classified all the data, just as some computers have been programmed to do, and the solution was in his brain, ready to use in the morning. "I go to bed with problems unsolved," Williams once explained, "but when I get up in the morning after having this quiet hour, the best solution I can devise inevitably comes to me."

If you want to find easy, resourceful answers to your current problems, you can practice your own version of this age-old presleep technique. After a bath and just before going to bed, think for a minute, and on a pad kept by your bedside, write down a problem you have been pondering in one sentence. Take time to make it crystal clear. This problem might be one of the concerns you discovered during your worry time, or it might be something else that popped into your mind. If the question you have written is simple and clear, the answer may come to you first thing in the morning, or it may take several days. But it will emerge. During sleeptime, your brain sorts through all possible solutions to problems.

The question must be one that can have a practical answer. As examples of possible solutions to presleep questions, here are some that have occurred to various friends about making their morning routine more harmonious. One family was nervous and irritable about using the bathroom in the morning. The father worked out a bathroom schedule and persuaded the pokiest of the kids to take a bath at night, rather than a shower in the morning. Breakfast time was pure hell for another friend. Her sleeping mind came up with a series of simple, effective solutions: "In order for me to expedite breakfast, I have to plan it the night before. Each night before I go to sleep I set the breakfast table, even putting all nonrefrigerated items on the table. I can save ten minutes each morning by putting the coffee and water in an electric coffeemaker that turns itself on at 6:30 A.M." Another friend described the morning as a battlefield of indecision in which everyone hunted for clean underwear and couldn't make up their minds about what to wear. She decided to have everyone set out their wardrobe the night before.

Reconditioning Therapy for Intractable Insomnia

Dr. Richard Bootzin's Stimulus Control Therapy is a highly regarded sleep-retraining technique which works for many common cases of insomnia. Specialists note the therapy may be difficult for the first few days of the regimen, but it has worked on hundreds of patients throughout the country, with results within two to three weeks. Dr. Peter Hauri of the Mayo Clinic says most chronic insomniacs can be retrained with the Bootzin method, eventually learning to sleep the instant their head hits the pillow.

GOING TO BED	WHAT TO DO IF YOU CAN'T SLEEP	TIME ELEMENT
Go to bed in the evening when tired.	If you don't fall asleep within 10 minutes, get out of bed. Walk out of the bedroom. Do any repetitive, boring task that is not a lot of fun: knitting, embroidery, needlepoint, solitaire or memorizing verbs in a foreign language.	Go back to bed when you feel you can go right to sleep.
Repeat this pattern of getting up in ten minutes if you can't fall asleep.	Repeat boring tasks.	Use an alarm clock to wake up at the time you need to get up each morning.
Never take a nap during the day.		

Appendix:
The Sleep/Temperament Connection
in Children

People in all societies once lived in strong groups of extended families. They were able to learn of life, loving, even parenting by observing others in the family. Unfortunately, this model has disappeared. To prevent early sleep and life clashes between children and parents, pediatric specialists at Arizona State College in Tempe worked out a remarkable program of temperament intervention. Its approach should be replicated worldwide. The program, Temperament Intervention for Parents Study (TIPS), is conducted under the supervision of Dr. Nancy Melvin, professor of nursing, and pediatric nurses Shirley Rees-McGee and Diana Jacobson. At TIPS, teams of nurses visit families and help young parents invent new strategies for dealing with bedtime, mealtime, getting dressed and whining. "One way to understand why a child disobeys is to think of behavior problems as a symptom of the 'fit' between a parenting approach and a child's temperament," says Professor Melvin. The nurses make sure that parents comprehend that there is no such thing as "one-size fits all parenting" and that the very way a child fusses and complains may be a demonstration of innate personality and not necessarily an interaction problem with a parent.

The TIPS program has devised a number of interesting categories for awareness of temperament. I'm not sure that I totally agree with all the criteria and conclusions the Arizona nurses have worked out, but just being aware of possible differences between a child's inborn temperament and the parents' temperaments may provide invaluable insights into potential life, behavior and sleep problems. Once you check for these traits you might have an "Aha!" and make some of the following observations:

- "It's not just that this kid is trying to foil me and roil me, but he has an inborn style and personal approach."
- "No, she is not a monster, but her physical energy is different from mine."
- "He is not a 'pest,' but is sensitive to (whatever)."

(Solutions to the many kinds of sleep problems related to the following categories are provided in the At-a-Glance Charts at the end of Chapters 5 and 6.)

1. MOOD: How does your child view the world? Some children see it as a friendly, pleasant place, while others see it as unpleasant. Positive, high-mood children view the world with rosy glasses and see the good side of events and people. Obviously, children who view the world this way are not distrustful and have an easier time falling asleep. Negative, low-mood children tend to be both pessimistic and realistic in evaluating life around them. These children also tend to cry more often. Viewing the world as an unpleasant place may make the child worry about trivial as well as real encounters and events, and this may show up in worried, fragmented sleep.

2. PREDICTABILITY OF RHYTHM: Children have either regular or irregular rhythms in terms of sleep, eating and elimination. Children who are highly regular have predictable rhythms and are quite comfortable in latching on to new schedules. These children will probably have an easy time developing their own strong sleep patterns. Children with irregular rhythms will get tired and hungry at different times of the day. Or it is also possible that children can start out in life with irregular master clock mechanisms. Since sleep is dependent on signals from one's internal clock, it may have turned night into day and vice versa in these children.

3. ADAPTABILITY: Have you noticed how much time your child needs to adjust to people, activities and new events? Does slowness in adaptability influence his or her ability to go to sleep easily and without a fuss? Children who are fast to adapt are cooperative and compliant so they are not so likely to have their night's sleep upset. However, children who are slow to adapt might be uncomfortable with anything new. Thus a new event or a new person in the family circle—certainly a new babysitter or daycare center—might present a problem at sleeptime. According to TIPS' experts, slow adapters tend to act stubborn, strong-willed and headstrong. This is

most useful information and should influence your parenting strategies, especially how you encourage a child to go to sleep.

4. PHYSICAL ENERGY OR ACTIVITY: How do you evaluate your child's activity level? Is it high, low or in between? Children with high energy or activity levels often get fidgety when asked to sit still and feel restless on days they have to stay inside. They are also prone to act impulsively. A high-energy level may mean lots of movement during the day. This will always make a child or adult happily tired for sleep. On the other hand, if there is too much nervous energy, this child may have a hard. time calming down in time for sleep. Restless and fidgety children should always be given long, serene, easy-does-it baths, consistent, calming herbal teas and long, loving bedtime stories.

Children with low energy or activity levels tend to move at a slower pace and prefer inactive pastimes, such as coloring, playing quietly with toys or watching TV. However, this lack of physical exertion may negatively influence their ability to fall asleep fast. Strategies for such a child might include a pre- or postsupper walk, possibly one including nature observation. All children, but these, in particular, need lots of fresh air streaming into the room as they sleep. This is true even in cold climates. A cover made with down feathers (which may provoke allergies in some children) is nevertheless a time-honored aid to sleep because the down adjusts to the needs of the body for more or less warmth. (To avoid potential allergy from the feathers, enclose down in two closely woven cotton duvets, and only take the top cover off to wash it.)

5. APPROACH TO LIFE: How does your child confront such new experiences as foods, people and being in an entirely new or unusual place? Approaching children tend to leap right into every new experience. But even though such a child may welcome new experiences, if the situation sours or is not success-ful, this may slightly influence a night's sleep. Withdrawing children hold back cautiously until they feel comfortable. If the event was not satisfactory or the comfort zone not met, that may more strongly influence a night's sleep pattern. If you think your child tends to be withdrawn and has a sudden change in sleep patterns, quietly check into the week's events so you can examine and confront difficult situations out loud.

6. PERSISTENCE: How does a child respond when something becomes diffi-cult? High-persistence children keep at a task even when it is above their skill level. Low-persistence children become easily frustrated. When con-fronted with something different or difficult, such children either ask for help immediately or abandon the project. Children who consistently aban-don projects eventually develop low self-esteem, and though never voicing

it aloud, they may tend to think of themselves as failures. This is often reflected in difficult sleep patterns.

For children with low-persistence levels, parents can recall personal incidents from their own life in which they overcame difficult situations by being determined and tenacious. Your child will never forget these object lessons, especially if they're not in the form of lectures, but anecdotes about life. If grandparents are alive, ask them for some of their own experiences in persistence. When they visit get them to tell these stories as part of storytelling about their own life or the lives of their parents or grandparents. Incorporate their stories into your storytelling times. If personal stories aren't available, you can always develop a personalized scenario like the one in Chapter 6 (under My Child Insists on Sleeping in Our Bed Every Night) or personalize the famous children's story, *The Little Engine That Could.*

7. DISTRACTIBILITY: Is your child easily distracted by something around him or her? Children with a high threshold for concentration are able to focus on what they are doing and are rarely diverted from it. Children with low thresholds for concentration are easily distracted, have a short attention span and are easily sidetracked from activities. These children need especially pleasant, firm, going-to-bed rituals. It is possible that such children will be easier to woo from sleep if there is unexpected household noise, outside traffic or light sifting into the room as they go to sleep or in the early morning. Low-level computer learning games are excellent aids in step-by-step thinking. They also lead to success, a very important element in an easily distracted child's life.

8. SENSORY THRESHOLD: How sensitive is your child to the five senses of touch, taste, smell, hearing and vision? A child with a high-sensory threshold is able to ignore such stimuli as noise, too much light, funny smells, the taste of a new food and can even wear clothes that are too tight or have an itchy label. A child with a low-sensory threshold will quickly and easily react to such discomforts. Sleep of sensory-sensitive children will probably be affected by such seemingly slight things as low-level noise, light from a street lamp, smells from a nearby restaurant, a new food, stiff bedclothes or any material that feels itchy. Such a child may also be sensitive to a household or neighborhood application of mosquito spray, the discharge from a new carpet or even the smell of leather in a new car. Once these things are noted, discussed or dispensed with, the child can probably sleep more easily and for longer periods of time.

9. EMOTIONAL SENSITIVITY: How do you rate your child in her mad, glad and sad moments? Is he emotionally sensitive or relatively insensitive? Are

his emotions accessible to him or hidden away? How do the emotions of fear, sorrow, hurt, embarrassment, worry or compassion influence your child's ability to fall asleep? Do worries or perceived problems arise during sleep as bad dreams, nightmares, night terrors or bedwetting? Can you gauge if a distracted sleep state is related to daytime reactions and emotional states?

The scenario section in Chapter 6 discusses various ways of dealing with a variety of daytime problems, how to listen to and then disarm a child's normal or powerful fears and worries. Keep in mind that bad dreams can be redreamed aloud in daylight. When you encourage a child to redream a frightening episode, the child learns to confront and overcome fears. This child may also need more reassurance than others.

Resources

Products

800 NUMBERS

Abra (organic bath salts; call for nearest distributor), 800-745-0761
Body Shop (bath and body products), 800-541-2535
Boericke & Tafel (homeopathy products), 800-876-9505
Boiron (homeopathy products), 1-800-BLUTUBE
Caswell Massey (general, old-fashioned body aids catalog), 800-326-0500
Dr. Singha's Mustard Bath (perfect for foot bath), 800-856-2862
Harney and Sons, Ltd. (special teas including chamomile flowers), 800-TEATIME
Heritage Store (new age remedies and products), 800-726-2232
Hickey Pharmacy (nutritional and homeopathic products), 800-724-5566
Luyties Pharmacal Co. (homeopathy and tissue salts), 800-325-8080
Nelson Bach USA Ltd. (homeopathic and Bach flower remedies), 800-314-BACH
Standard Homeopathic Co. (tissue salts), 800-624-9659
Vitamin Shoppe (supplements and remedies), 800-223-1216
Walnut Acres (organic food shopping by mail), 800-433-3998
Weleda (Orris root sticks and other excellent natural products), 800-421-1030
Willner Chemists (nutritional products), 800-545-1106

ACUPRESSURE SLEEP PRODUCTS

Self Care Catalog
5850 Shellmound St.

Emeryville, CA 94608-1901
Phone: 800-345-3371
E-mail: slfcare@aol.com
A prime source of preventive medicine products, including a variety of
that promote sleep: (1) Adhesive wrist patches to press on sleep acupuncture points. Claims they need only be used nightly for two weeks to
establish long-term improvement in sleep. (2) Soft divided rubber globe
called "Still Point" is placed under the skull to produce gentle pressure
which relaxes the nervous system.

ALLERGY-FREE BEDDING AIDS

Heart of Vermont
P.O. Box 612
Barre, VT 05641
Phone: 800-639-4123
Organic wool or cotton innerspring mattresses and boxspring sets, mattress
pad, barrier cloth mattress protectors with zipper; carbonized (natural process cleaning) wool items; organic flannel and chambray sheets, pillow
cases, comforters; organic baby receiving blankets, crib sheets and pillowcases. Also platform and Mission hardwood beds.

KB Cotton Pillows, Inc.
P.O. Box 57
DeSoto, TX 75123
Phone: 800-544-3752
Turn-of-the-century 100% cotton pillows with 100% removable cotton
ticking prewashed and rinsed in baking powder solution to make chemical
free. Available in variety of small to larger standard sizes.

Nontoxic Environments, Inc.
P.O. Box 384
Newmarket, NH 03857
Information: 603-659-5919
Phone orders: 800-789-4348
Fax: 603-659-5933
Large building, household and personal product catalog for the chemically
sensitive and earthwise person. A doctor's prescription is required for in-
surance coverage for organic cotton mattresses, futons and mattress pads.
All manner of nontoxic items include cotton and wool pillows; wool mat-
tress pads and comforters (with cotton covers); and organic cotton baby
items for sleep and playing.

Priorities
70 Walnut St.
Wellesley, MA 02181
Phone: 800-553-5398
Allergy-free box springs and mattresses; mattress covers, comforters, pillows and pillow covers to protect people with dust allergies or asthma. A wide variety of other allergy-protection products, including dust mite sprays; air, window and water filters; safe shampoo for cats and dogs; and an antidander spray for cats, dogs or birds.

Self Care Catolog (see complete listing under Acupressure Sleep Products)
Phone: 800-345-3371
The adjustable wood frame Natura Total Sleep System with adjustable head rest, lumbar support and leg lift as well as a series of narrow mattress pads and cotton duvets. "Medibed" anti-allergy mattress, pillow, duvet and barrier cotton protectors.

Seventh Generation
1 Mill Street, Box A26
Burlington, VT 05401-1530
Phone: 800-456-1177
Fax: 800-456-1139
Natural fiber sheets, towels, activeware, sleepwear; cotton throws; linen and cotton sheets; lightweight large sleep mask of "GreenCotton;" aromatherapy sleep mask; a unique, quiet electrostatic air filter window fan; and allergy-free American West style jute throw rugs. The catalog contains hundreds of products for healthy personal, home and planet-friendly use. (The organization takes its name from one of the laws of the Iroquois: "In our every deliberation, we must consider the impact of our decisions on the next seven generations.")

BED BOARDS AND BEDDING FOR BAD BACKS

BackSaver Products Company
53 Jeffery Ave.
Holliston, MA 01746
Phone: 800-251-2225
Fax: 800-443-9609
Specializes in "BackSaver" chairs, writing desks and bedding equipment. The chairs all have support and high-function aids, including temperature-sensitive and self-adjusting "Wonder Foam." Bedding aids include "Comfort Pad" to support the lower back while sleeping; "Wonder Foam" mattress top that claims to eliminate painful pressure points and increase

circulation; pregnancy-support pillow and knee cushion; high support bed-reading pillow; hypoallergenic neck pillow, which is described as cervical spine support to prevent neck and back pain. Several people have told me the products were worth their steep price.

The Vermont Country Store
P.O. Box 3000
Manchester Center, VT 05255
Phone: 802-362-2400
If you can't have a bedboard made to the right size by a local carpenter, you can order a folding bedboard that comes 59 inches long and in two widths: 24 inches and 30 inches. For a twin bed, order one 30 inches; for a double bed, order two 24 inches; for queen and king size beds, order two 30 inches.

BEDWETTING
One Step Ahead
P.O. Box 517
Lake Bluff, IL 60044
Phone: 800-274-8440
Protective children's bed pad that absorbs 6 cups of liquid.

Self Care Catalog (see complete listing under Acupressure Sleep Products)
Phone: 800-345-3371
"DryTime for Bedwetting" is a moisture sensor that wakes up deep sleepers with a loud alarm. Claims the child eventually learns to respond to bladder signals without the alarm, thus eliminating bedwetting problems.

Vermont Country Store (see complete listing under Bed Boards)
Phone: 802-362-2400
Full waterproof pad with cotton flannel top for all size beds.

BOOKS
The Bach Flower Remedies by Nora Weeks & Victor Bullen (London: C.W. Daniels Company Ltd.).

The Encylopedia of Sleep and Dreaming by Mary A. Carskadon, Ph.D., ed. (New York: Macmillan).

Handbook of the Bach Flower Remedies by Phillip M. Chancelor (New Canaan, Conn.: Keats).

The Medical Discoveries of Edward Bach Physician by Nora Weeks, C.W. (London: Daniel Company Ltd.).

Narcolepsy Primer by Meeta Goswami, M.P.H., Ph.D. and Michael J. Thorpy, M.D. (Bronx, N.Y.: Montefiore Medical Center).

Nighttime Parenting: How to Get Your Baby and Child to Sleep by William Sears, M.D. (New York: Plume/La Leche League International Book).

No More Sleepless Nights by Peter Hauri, Ph.D. and Shirley Linde, Ph.D. (New York: John Wiley & Sons).

Principles and Practice of Sleep Medicine, 2d ed. (New York: Saunders).

Restful Sleep by Deepak Chopra, M.D. (New York: Harmony Books).

Solve Your Child's Sleep Problems by Richard Ferber, M.D. (New York: Simon & Schuster).

Some Must Watch While Some Must Sleep by William Dement, M.D., Ph.D. (New York: Norton).

The Terrific, No Tears Bedtime Book by Marjorie R. Nelsen (Longwood, Fla.: Partners In Learning, Inc.). A child's bedtime routine with a beginning and no-tears ending for ages 2-6 years. Mrs. Nelson also conducts early childhood and parent education classes (write to: Partners In Learning, Inc., 1417 Noble St., Longwood, FL 32750; phone and fax: 407-831-2947).

Waking Up Dry: How to End Bedwetting Forever by Martin Scharf, Ph.D. (Cincinnati: Writer's Digest Books).

BREATHING DEVICES
Self Care Catalog (see complete listing under Acupressure Sleep Products)
Phone: 800-345-3371
Air-cooled steam device called "Therapeutic Steam Inhaler" relieves parched throats, respiratory congestion, coughs and allergy problems.

CHILDREN'S BATH AIDS
One Step Ahead (complete listing under Bedwetting)
Phone: 800-274-8440
Baby tubs include unique contoured bath cushion that fits in sink or tub, marvelous for newborn; "safety" plastic tub designed to fit children from 0 to 6 months and, when turned over, from 6 months to 2 years; inflatable baby tub that fits into the larger bathtub. Bath seat, with suction cups, folds and opens on the front. Knee aid, nifty foam padded vinyl mat,

protect adults' knees and arms while bathing baby in tub. Hair washing aid for toddler sends water from bath through "hippo spout."

CHILDREN'S SLEEP AIDS
One Step Ahead (complete listing under Bedwetting)
Phone: 800-274-8440
I like this catalog company because the products are all tested and enormously useful. Their Baby Bjorn Infant Carrier, which can be used from one week to ten months, is the best. Many sleep aids include: a gentle, automatic dimming light that goes from light to dark in a fifteen-minute interval; knitted cotton bassinet and crib bedding in mellow and vivid colors; a lambskin fleece throw for the baby to sleep on; burp pads; flotation sleeping devices, which are said to be cooler in the summer and warmer in the winter; baby-sized adjustable headrests; a variety of safe infant sleep bumpers to keep the baby sleeping on its side or back; a crib rocker that responds to a baby's cries; an easily mounted crib cassette-player with nightlight that plays tapes of the womb, sleep-inducing sounds of nature and lullabies; protective bed-wetting pads; toddler-sized pillows and cases; a zippered "Cozy Crib Tent" for toddler who tries to climb out of crib. Nursing aids for the mother include holders for one child or twins, breast pumps, sterile milk collection bags and foot stool.

SleepTight
4710 East Walnut St.
Westerville, OH 43081
Phone: 800-NO-COLIC (800-662-6542)
Device calms colicky babies and reduces crying. Invented by a father with a colicky baby, device is attached to the crib and mimics the soothing rocking and sound of a car traveling at 55 miles an hour with closed windows. In some cases, device is covered by insurance under the code 789.0 (abdominal pain and infantile colic).

Toys R Us
"Prop A Baby" is an inexpensive, effective "bumper"-type enveloping pillow that encases the baby and helps it sleep on its side or back. "Prop A Baby Deluxe" contains microchip that reproduces the comforting swish-swish sounds fetus heard in mother's womb. Store doesn't sell this mail order, but it is shown in the crib section of the 1996 store catalog.

DAYLIGHT & SUNLIGHT APPLIANCES
Light appliances can help retrain body to adopt normal sleep patterns. They should be used with advice and help from sleep professionals, but they are available to the general public through the following mail order houses:

Northern Light Technologies
8971 Henri Bourassa West
St. Laurent, Quebec, Canada HE 1P7
Phone: 800-236-0066
Local: 514-335-1763
Desk lamp, designed to bring spring and summer light levels into home or office during winter days, provides diffuse light without heat.

Self Care Catalog (for complete listing see Acupressure Sleep Products)
Phone: 800-345-3371
Sunrise clock that awakens sleepers with gradual, refreshing daylight simulation.

The SunBox Company
19217 Orbit Dr.
Gaithersburg, MD 20879
Phone: 800-LITE-YOU (800-548-3968)
Local: 301-869-5980
Fax: 301-977-2281
Original manufacturer of light units offers UV-free warrantied, small and large, standing and portable light boxes, light visors, dawn-to-dusk light simulators, full-spectrum fluorescents and incandescent bulbs to correct sleep disorders, body clock disturbances, winter blues, SAD (Seasonal Affective Disorder), jet lag, shift worker body clock disturbances and menstrual irregularities. Also, offers excellent list of books on light therapy, winter blues, jet lag and body rhythms.

Vitamin Shoppe
Phone: 800-223-1216
National chain has big, reliable catalog of all kinds of natural items. For instance, carries famed Finnish Chromolux full-spectrum light bulbs that duplicate natural daylight indoors and offer the lowest price in the country (as of March 1997). Since they provide true color of natural sunlight, I buy these bulbs in bulk. While each is expensive compared with usual supermarket bulbs, they last for 3,500 hours. Use them over work areas, desk, in kitchen, wherever you sit and read. A must for anyone who dreads dark, dim days of winter or feels depressed in January and February. While

they can't accomplish what lux lights (five times the strength of ordinary lights) can, they can certainly help avoid some of the winter blahs and may contribute to better winter sleeping as they uplift the spirits.

HERBAL OUTLETS
Aphrodisia
264 Bleeker St.
New York, NY 10014
Phone: 212-989-6440
Dried herbs, potpourri.

Earth's Essence
28 Chester Turnpike
Auburn, NH 03032
100 herbal products, books, videos; catalog $2.

Gaia Botanicals
Box 8485
Philadelphia, PA 19101
$5 for 100-page catalog of 800 herbs and spices, including Chinese and Ayurvedic books.

R. Hartenthaler
133 Henderson
Norwood, PA 19074
Bulk medicinal and culinary herbs, essential oils, books; catalog $1 refunded with first order.

Health Center for Better Living
6189 Taylor Rd.
Naples, FL 33942
Phone: 941-566-2611
Medical herbs in eight forms.

Herb and Spice Collection
P.O. Box 118
Norway, IA 52318
Phone: 800-786-1388
160-page catalog listing 5,000 products; $2 refunded with order.

Homestead Herbs
2223 Cold Springs La.
Spring Garden, CA 95971
Dream pillows, potpourri, sachets, teas.

Indiana Botanic Gardens Herbalist
P.O. Box 5
Hammond, IN 46325
Phone: 219-949-4040
Famous old catalog of herbal products.

Sierra
P.O. Box 412
Kinderhook, NY 12106
Phone: 800-695-2349

HERBS: ORGANIC
Blessed Herbs (wildcrafted and organic dried herbs)
Rt. 5, Box 1042
Ava, MO 65608
Phone: 417-683-5721

Dry Creek Herb Farm
13035 Dry Creek Rd.
Auburn, CA 95602
Phone: 916-878-2441

Great Lakes Herb Company (also bath products; catalog $1)
P.O. Box 6713
Minneapolis, MN 55406

Terra Firma Botanicals, Inc.
126 Sutherlin La.
Eugene, OR 95405
Wildcrafted and organic herbal products, fresh and dried herbal extracts,
flower oils, skin salves, massage oils. Catalog $1 refunded with first order.

HOT WATER BOTTLES & ALTERNATIVES
Self Care Catolog (see complete listing under Acupressure Sleep Products)
Phone: 800-345-3371
"Angel Turtle" is an all-natural alternative to a stiff hot water bottle; con-

tains flax seed and polenta grains covered with washable cotton/linen. Two or three minutes in a microwave will give you half hour of soft, flexible warmth.

Vermont Country Store (see complete listing under Bed Boards)
Phone: 802-362-2400
Offers thick-skinned British bottle with soothing, removable 100% cotton chamois jacket which helps retain heat. In cold climates use to warm children's and adults' feet; will comfort a crying baby.

INCONTINENCE
One Step Ahead (see complete listing under Bedwetting)
Phone: 800-274-8440
Bed pad holds up to 6 cups of liquid and protects a child's mattress from bed-wetting accidents.

Self Care Catolog (see complete listing under Acupressure Sleep Products)
Phone: 800-345-3371
Carries the following aids: "HealthDri" panties and underwear for men and women; Kegel vaginal weights to strengthen women's pelvic floor; bedwetting alarm device for children.

LAMP THAT REDUCES STRESS
Whole Life Products
1334 Pacific Ave.
Forest Grove, OR 97116
Phone: 800-634-9057
Antistress lamp projection duplicates an entire full-spectrum 6-foot rainbow without brightening room. Said to ease stress and help relaxation and sleep.

LIGHTS (full-spectrum daylight bulbs; see also Daylight/Sunlight Appliances)
Seventh Generation, 800-456-1139
Vitamin Shoppe, 800-223-1216
Walnut Acres, 800-433-3998

MASKS FOR SPECIAL EFFECTS
Whole Life Products (complete listing under Lamp That Reduces Stress)

Phone: 800-634-9057
Two available: (1) "NovaDreamer," which comes with instructions on lucid dreaming techniques, is lightweight eye mask with an enclosed micro chip that recognizes rapid eye movements (REM) during dreams. The chip gives a flash to help you be aware that you are dreaming. Once alterted, you can participate in the dream process. (2) StressShield goggles block outside light and bathe the eyes in uniform light field and color to help you meditate and become calm.

MISCELLANEOUS MAIL ORDER CATALOGS
Hickey Pharmacy
888 2nd Ave.
New York, NY 10017
Phone: 800-724-5566
Pharmacist Jerry Hickey has extensive knowledge of nutrition and alternative therapies.

Willner Chemists, Nutritional Supplement Professionals
100 Park Ave.
New York, NY 10017
Orders: 800-633-1106
Fax: 212-545-0951
http://www.Willner.com
Reliable nutritional supplement company that carries variety of international and national homeopathic manufacturers and tissue salt products. Excellent nutritional pharmacists and other staff are geared to national as well as international mail order services.

NIGHT LIGHTS
Earth Care Catalog
555 Leslie St.
Ukiah, CA 95482-5507
Phone: 800-347-0070
Flat, attractive, plug-in night lights are sometimes hard to buy at neighborhood hardware stores. Carries cool light in triangular design with these advantages: built-in outlet (which means you don't lose an outlet!), lifetime guarantee, costs only 5 cents a year to run. Two other interesting sleep-aid items: battery light that is mounted on wall or sits on table; high-tech, long, flexible-neck halogen light for night-owl reader.

One Step Ahead (complete listing under Bedwetting)

Phone: 800-274-8440

Three-in-one nursery light that plugs into wall as night light or can be unplugged to become flashlight or long-lasting emergency light in case power goes off. Also, "Autofade Bedside Light" (handsome table light) fades from bright to dim to dark over fifteen minutes; helps infants adjust to dark and equates restful sleep with darkness.

NURSING AIDS

Two marvelous inventions have been patented, and perhaps by the time you read this, they will be manufactured. (1) Patent number 5,571,084 by William Palmer is modern adjustable "flak vest" that contains micro-chip vacuum pump. Chip allows woman to program pumping of breast milk to accommodate her body and imitate action of baby's suckling. "The object is to get the most milk in the shortest time," says Palmer. (2) Patent number 5,573,153 by Penny Stillman is shoulder cloth that holds bottle at right angle for nursing.

PILLOWS THAT SUPPORT BODY, NECK, EYES
Dreamtime
343 Soquel Ave., Suite 271
Santa Cruz, CA 95062
Phone: 408-464-6702
Fax: 408-464-6703

All-size sleeping pillows, sachets, eye pillows and meditation cushions filled with organic buckwheat hulls to conform to head, neck and forehead to provide "passive, contoured support." Sleeping pillows are 100% cotton; eye pillowcases are pure Oriental silk. Eye pillow provide gentle, soothing acupressure on eye muscles, ideal for napping and meditating. One aroma-therapy sachet, which contains mugwort combined with lavender and chamomile, is said to reduce insomnia and enhance dreaming.

Healthware 2 Bodycare Company
610 22nd St., Suite 247
San Francisco, CA 94107
Phone: 800-829-6560
Local: 415-626-7378
Fax: 415-626-7803

"Rest Assured" dream and neck pillows; "Rest your eyes, temple, head and forehead" pillow filled with lightweight, durable buckwheat hulls which hold their molded shape in silk or cotton covers. Very relaxing.

Self Care Catalog (see complete listing under Acupressure Sleep Products)
Phone: 800-345-3371
Pillows for back, cervical, whole body support, reading pain-free, "Dr. Riter's Ease Neck and Shoulder Relaxer."

Smart Support, Inc.
634-C North Poplar St.
Orange, CA 92668
Phone: 800-745-5692 (800-PILLOW2)
"Self-Adjustable Neck Support" pillow developed by physician specializing in arthritis. Hotter/colder neck collars in small, medium, large sizes.

SLEEP MASKS
Key Enterprises
80 Austin Dr, #111
Burlington, VT 05401
Phone: 802-865-3063
Cotton sleep mask and aromatherapy sleep mask (lavender and balsam to relieve congestion) block light and help produce natural melatonin. "I-Rest: A Pillow for the Eye" is 100% cotton velvet bag filled with herbs and rice that is said to be easy on the mind, sinuses and eyes, especially when computer-strained.

Whole Life Products (complete listing under Lamp That Reduces Stress)
Phone: 800-634-9057

SLEEP TAPES
One Step Ahead (complete listing under Bedwetting)
Phone: 800-274-8440
Tapes for infants that duplicate white noise sounds from nature or those of mother's womb. Also, tape machine that can be attached to crib.

"The Sleep Tape," video issued by Simon & Schuster
Ask for at local store that sells videos.
Tips for relaxation, sleep rituals and nature scenes backed by soothing piano music.

SNORING AIDS
Self Care Catalog (complete listing under Acupressure Sleep Products)
Phone: 800-345-3371

Five products: (1) "Therapuetic Steam Inhaler" provides air-cooled steam to ease congestion. (2) "BreatheEZ" clip stimulates septum nerve to open up congested nasal passages. (3) "Nozovent" is flexible piece of plastic that widens nostrils and helps increase air flow. (4) "Snore-No-More" are herbal tablets that open breathing passages. (5) "Side Rester Pillow" encourages user to sleep on side (snorer should not sleep on back).

I came across the following two professional sources while at the annual American Sleep Disorders Association Conference. The first must be obtained through a dentist, the other through a physician or sleep clinic.

The Hebst Appliance
Great Lakes Orthodontics, Ltd.
199 Fire Tower Dr.
Tonawanda, NY 14150
Adjustable appliance helps control snoring, sleep apnea and malocclusions in children. Soft version similar to an athletic mouthguard.

TheraSnore Appliance
Phone: 800-477-6673
Said to be ideal for patients who cannot or will not tolerate CPAP appliances and/or have failed surgery; said to take only one night to adjust to.

TINCTURES
Widely available by mail and at local health stores. Nature's Answer provides nonalcoholic tincture; call 800-645-5720 to obtain name of seller nearest you.

TISSUE SALTS
Available in local health food stores and from many sources through the mail.

Luyties Pharmacal Co., NuAge Laboratories Ltd.
4200 Laclede Ave.
St. Louis, MO 63108
Phone: 800-325-8080
Outside U.S.A.: 314-533-9660
Homeopathic tissue salts in a travel kit manufactured by old homeopathic company.

TRYPTOPHAN

The useful sleep-inducing amino acid L-tryptophan is no longer available over-the-counter but must be prescribed by a physician. Usually the prescribing physician orders this through members of the International Association of Compounding Pharmacists. For a local referral, call, fax or browse the Internet.

International Association of Compounding Pharmacists
Box 1365
Sugar Land, TX 77487
Phone: 800-927-4227
Local: 713-933-8400
Fax: 713-495-0602
Internet: http://www.iacp.com/iacp

WHITE NOISE MACHINES

If you are bothered by street sounds, barking dogs, snoring or inner ear noises, white noise machines often help overcome the problem. The sounds they produce vary from nature to neutral sounds designed to lull you to sleep.

One Step Ahead (complete listing Bedwetting)
Phone: 800-272-8440

Whole Life Products (complete listing under Lamp That Reduces Stress)
Phone: 800-634-9057
Plug-in or battery-operated machine called "LifeSounds" produces six anti-stress, sleep-inducing sounds. Three are for colicky babies, children or adults with sleeping problems: one duplicates, via ultrasound, what fetus heard in the womb; another mother's heartbeat; another guitar lullabies. Other white sounds are of brook, rain and surf.

Services

ALTERNATIVE MEDICAL/THERAPEUTIC ORGANIZATIONS

American Association of Naturopathic Physicians
2366 Eastlake Ave. E., Suite 322
Seattle, WA 98102
Phone: 206-323-7610

American Association of Oriental Medicine (acupuncture)
433 Front St.
Catasauqua, PA 18032
Phone: 610-433-2448

American Chiropractic Association
1701 Clarendon Bvld.
Arlington, VA 22209
Phone: 800-968-4636

American Holistic Medical Association
4101 Lake Boone Trail, Suite 201
Raliegh, NC 27607
Phone: 909-787-5181

The Ayurvedic Institute
P.O. Box 23445
Albuquerque, NM 87192
Phone: 505-291-9698

Homeopathic Educational Services
2124 Kittredge St.
Berkeley, CA 94704
Phone: 510-649-0294

International Chiropractic Association
1110 Glebe Rd., Suite 1000
Arlington, VA 22201
Phone: 800-423-4690

National Center for Homeopathy
801 N. Fairfax St., Suite 306
Alexandria, VA 22314
Phone: 703-548-7790

BODY WORK ORGANIZATIONS
American Massage Therapy Association
820 Davis St., Suite 100
Evanston, IL 60201
Phone: 847-864-0123

Feldenkreis Guild
524 Ellswortyh St.
P.O. Box 489
Albany, OR 97321
Phone: 800-775-2118

Trager Institute
21 Locust Ave.
Mill Valley, CA 94941
Phone: 415-388-2688

The Upledger Institute
11211 Prosperity Farms Rd.
Palm Beach Gardens, FL 33410
Phone: 800-233-5880

MISCELLANEOUS SUPPORT GROUPS

The American Narcolepsy Association
P.O. Box 1187
San Carlos, CA 94070
Phone: 800-327-6085

The International Network for Children and Families
P.O. Box 7236
Gainesville, FL 32605
Phone: 800-257-9002
Offers course called "Redirecting Children's Behavior."

Narcolepy Network
P.O. Box 190
Belmont, CA 94002
Phone: 415-591-7884

National Sleep Foundation,
122 South Robertson Blvd., 3rd floor
Los Angeles, CA 90048
Phone: 800-890-3222

Restless Legs Syndrome Foundation, Inc.
304 Glenwood Ave.
Raleigh, NC 27603
Twelve million people, or 5% of the population, are thought to have this sleep-deprivation syndrome or related syndromes of Periodic Leg Movement Disorder (PLMD) or Periodic Leg Movement During Sleep (PLMS), which also affects about 5% of the population. Included in membership in this nonprofit organization is a doctor referral program, publications, newsletter called *Night Walkers*, lists of local support groups and various services to patients, families and doctors.

PARENT INTERNET SUPPORT AND INFORMATION GROUPS
CYFERNET (articles on families and development)
http://www.mes.umn.edu/CYFERNET

ERIC Clearinghouse on Elementary and Early Childhood Education
(research and access to wide variety of education and developmental
information)
http://ericps.ed.uiuc.edu

Family Education Network
http:/families.com

National PTA (information on education and development)
http://www.pta.org

SLEEP DISORDER CENTERS
For list of accredited member sleep disorders centers near you, contact:

American Sleep Disorders Association
1610 14th St. NW, Suite 300
Rochester, MN 55901
Phone: 507-287-6006
Fax: 507-287-6008

Children's Sleep Disorders Center
4200 W. Peterson Ave.
Chicago, IL 60646
Phone: 708-368-6799

Index

pressure points, 150, 196–198
prostate problems, *see* incontinence
Pulsatilla, 127, 134, 176
  for fear of the dark, 109, 143
  for rocking needs, 105
  for separation anxiety, 111, 141,
    144, 146, 152
  for sleeplessness, 75, 151

ragweed, 168
rapid-eye movement, *see* REM
reconditioning techniques, *see*
  behavior modification
red pepper ointment, 20
relaxing exercises, 193–196
REM sleep, 9, 14
  see also dreams
rescue remedy, 180
restless leg syndrome, 23–28, 116
  see also muscle twitch; periodic
    leg movement disorder
restless sleep, 77, 109
restlessness, 165–166
retinitis pigmentosa, 82
Reye's syndrome, 21
rheumatoid arthritis, 82
rhythms, 202
RLS, *see* restless leg syndrome
rocking to sleep, 103–105,
  126–127, 139
room temperature, 60–61, 96,
  106–107
rosemary, 171

safety precautions
  with night terrors, 124–125
  with sleep walking, 123
sage, 172
salt rub, 187
San-yin-chiao point, 197
Schuessler, William, 177–178

screaming, 109
scullcap, 167
seasonal affective disorder, 51–54
sensitivity, 204–205
sensory threshold, 204
separation anxiety, 111, 134, 144
Shen-man point, 196
shift work, 16, 48–49
shock, 144, 154
shoulder stretch, 195
SIDS (sudden infant death
  syndrome), 97
silica
  for dreaming, 78, 141, 143
  for drowsiness, 111
  for jerking limbs, 28, 117
  for pain, 78
  for sleepiness, 146
  for sleeplessness, 75
  for sleepwalking, 141
  for yawning, 119
sinus infection, 142
sleep
  and age, 7–8, 17
  conference on, 6
  and memory, 10
  nonrefreshing, 108, 146, 189
  process, 9–17
  resistance to, 55
  stages of, 9–11
    chart, 12–14
    in children, 121
    in infants, 90–95
  see also sleep disturbances; sleep
    habits
sleep apnea, 37–39, 83, 125
sleep contracts, 88, 157
sleep disturbances
  in adults, 5–8, 18–54, 72–84
  in children, 120–154
  homeopathic remedies for,
    175–177
  in infants, 96–119